A MORE DIFFICULT EXERCISE

A More Difficult Exercise

DIANA MORAN

BLOOMSBURY

First published 1989
Copyright © 1989 by Diana Moran

Bloomsbury Publishing Ltd. 2 Soho Square, London WIV 5DE

British Library Cataloguing in Publication Data

Moran, Diana
A more difficult exercise
1. Memoir
I. Title
613.7'092'4

ISBN 0-7475-0349-4

Typeset by Hewer Text Composition Services, Edinburgh
Printed in Great Britain by Butler & Tanner, Frome, Somerset

'On Friday, May 13 1988, I was given some news which was to turn my world upside down, disturbing not only my life but the lives of my close family and friends.

But its effects were to go deeper, forcing me to reassess my life and priorities. It was a very painful experience but from it I gained courage, strength and understanding. Through this time, I kept a detailed diary, a report of the day's happenings and my feelings and reactions to them. By publishing the contents of this very personal diary and the subsequent soul-searchings which accompanied it, I hope to inform and console some of the many thousands of women who are given similar news. I hope too it will help allay fear and confusion should well-meaning people confront them with old wives' tales and alternative treatments, and encourage them to decide for themselves what they want to happen so that they may be in charge of their own bodies.'

– Diana Moran

FOR WOMEN EVERYWHERE
TO DISPEL FEARS
AND ENCOURAGE VIGILANCE

CONTENTS

MAY

Friday, 13 May

The alarm sounds. It's eight o'clock and time to get up. Oh, my head! This is going to be an effort. But last night's Glamorous Granny competition at Butlin's in Bognor Regis was worth a bit of a hangover.

It was a most enjoyable evening alongside David Jacobs, as compere, and television and sports personalities Fred Dineage, Wincey Willis, Ray Reardon and Alan Ball. We judges felt we'd picked a good winner. She was lovely, aged forty-eight, slim and blonde with a beautiful smile. A market trader and mother of four, she had two grandchildren including a new-born baby. She certainly wasn't the traditional image of a gran – my own granny was wonderful, but she didn't look like that.

I dropped into bed exhausted at two o'clock this morning after being driven back from Sussex, leaving 'Glam Gran' enjoying the celebrations with her family and the other competitors. Bet she's got a bit of a headache as well this morning . . .

Nevertheless, it's time to show a leg. I've got a lot to do today. I have to put the finishing touches to some magazine articles, and I've also got to caption the pictures for the exercise section of a new keep-fit book that I've been asked to contribute to. But first I have an appointment to keep, so I'd better get moving. Punctually at nine the taxi arrives at my flat overlooking the Thames and takes me to the Fulham Road. At the reception desk of Granard House, part of the Royal Marsden Hospital, I'm greeted by cheery staff who ask me if I've been here before. I say no, but tell them I have an appointment with Mr Scott at ten o'clock and I'm early.

They ask me to register. Date – Friday the 13th. 'Hope you're not superstitious!' jokes the receptionist. 'Name?'

'Diana Moran.'

'Age?'

'Forty-eight.'

Finally, 'Next of kin?'

A lump comes to my throat as I reply, 'Timothy Moran, eldest son.' I swallow hard and get led to the nearby waiting room where all eyes turn on me, the latest stranger to be inspected.

The room is full of people anxiously flipping through magazines in an effort to avoid one another's eyes. I grab a magazine and do the same, but I'm conscious of some whispering going on in the far corner. Why do people think that others can't hear them and what they're secretly talking about? I feel like standing up and announcing: 'Yes, I *am* the Green Goddess,' to put them and myself out of our miseries. Glancing up, momentarily, the younger of the two women catches my eye and smiles. She turns triumphantly to her friend and says, 'Told you it was her.' I hear the nurse call my name and thankfully escape.

Mr Scott greets me kindly. It isn't the first time we've met. He asks me to sit down and tries to put me at my ease. Looking at his notes, he seems to be reaffirming his previous suspicions as he shuffles the X-rays and reports in front of him.

I decide to take the initiative. 'It's cancer, isn't it?'

He responds with a long, sad nod. 'I'm sorry I have to tell you the news you didn't want to hear.'

I'm stunned into silence, and fight for words. Mr Scott touches my arm reassuringly as I begin to search ridiculously and frantically for a hankie. He hands me a tissue and tactfully leaves the room for a minute.

I feel a sense of shock, combined with a strange awareness of the reality of the situation. My biggest fear of the last twenty years has finally become a reality. I've been so lucky until now. All the other lumps in my breasts – too many to recall – have been found after surgery to be benign. In fact I've become blasé about them. But now my luck has run out.

But no, it can't be true – I'm the keep-fit lady. Perhaps there's been a mistake. But if it *is* true, how will I cope? Or will I die? I begin to panic. Oh, my God, that's why they needed to know my next of kin! Tim and my other son, Nic, would be told first – and they don't know any of this. The thought appals me. Oh, dear God, no. Why me?

Mr Scott returns, shuts the door and sits down, pulling his chair closer to mine. He starts talking gently, but the words go in one ear and out the other. I can't digest any of it.

Suddenly I feel cold and alone. How will I manage? I've chosen independence. I've recently divorced. How will I pay the everyday bills, let alone the mortgage? I'll have to move. Who'll come and look after me? Who'll nurse me? I blurt out all my worries. Mr Scott lets me unburden myself on him and just quietly listens.

When I'm a little more controlled he tells me he's going to fill me in on some of the important details, so that I have all the information I need to make my decision. And he stresses that it *is* my decision – surgery will only be performed if I agree to it, though I should have the biopsy anyway to make certain. Even so, he will go ahead and make arrangements as if I am definitely going to go through with it – which is clearly what he recommends in his professional capacity – so that the waiting period is not prolonged unnecessarily. I would be in hospital for seven to ten days, and take six to eight weeks to recover. After that time my movement would be back to normal but I might lack energy.

He starts to explain the kind of operations that are performed for cancer of the breast. I have non-invasive cancer, he tells me, but unfortunately, despite its name, its treatment has to be more rigorous. Invasive cancer can consist of no more than a single lump, so that a lumpectomy rather than a complete mastectomy can be performed. My kind, non-invasive cancer, is more widely distributed – hence the need for a mastectomy.

To illustrate this, on the mammograms I had taken when I

last saw him he shows me the extent of the calcification within my left breast. These grains of salt look like stars to me, but he tells me they are probably indications of widespread intra-duct cancer. He tells me he's found some other nodules in my right breast – not the same, but also in need of surgery.

It just can't be happening to me. Not my right breast as well. I feel sick, but I try to control myself. I must find out more. I ask him how this can be – for twenty years I've been finding lumps, and for this reason have been sensible and have had regular six-monthly check-ups with a West Country surgeon. He saw me only two months ago and gave me the all-clear. And I've checked my breasts regularly myself and can feel nothing. Now Mr Scott is telling me I have cancer, and recommending a bilateral mastectomy. This surely has to be wrong, doesn't it?

Mr Scott is very calm and most understanding and tells me that the mammogram, an X-ray of the breast, shows up troublesome areas before they can be felt. This, he adds, is why I'm so lucky. Lucky? It certainly doesn't feel like it to me. But he assures me that I am, because the extent of the cancer is small enough to be operated on with a high rate of success. He takes some fluid from my breast for examination and asks me to go upstairs for a chest X-ray and some blood tests.

When I return he talks to me again. He realizes how important my physical health and appearance are to my work, and is therefore concerned as to how I'm going to feel about my looks after the operation. What looks? I think grimly. And I wonder if I will ever get back to my high standard of physical fitness. I have a vivid imagination, and I'm writing myself off rapidly. Next he asks me if I have a boyfriend. Rather sarcastically I reply: 'I did, but for how much longer I'm very doubtful.' What a sight I'm going to be – my work and no doubt my love life too at an end. I mentally dig a hole and begin to bury myself.

'So where do we go from here?' I ask him. He tells me he has decided to refer me to another surgeon, who may possibly be able to reconstruct my breasts at a later date. He draws a rough diagram showing how this might be done, but assures me it will look better than his drawing. I tell him I'll keep it to remind him he said so.

He keeps emphasizing that I mustn't think of myself as ill. I can see he's right in a way, and it's sensible psychology, but I'm going to have to keep convincing myself. Finally he refers to a letter he has received from my West Country surgeon, who was sent my details after my first visit a few weeks ago. I feel pleased and comforted that the two men have compared notes. Mr Scott advises me to go down and see him, on the assumption that I will want to have my treatment there. I realize this is medical ethics – he doesn't want to tread on another surgeon's toes. But my life is up here in London now, and in any case I'm not sure I could cope with the trauma of being in hospital in Bristol. My ex-husband lives there, and so do many members of my family with whom relationships have been strained since my divorce. Mr Scott seems to understand all this, and I'm so happy when he says he'll look after me here in London, if that's what I want.

As I leave, a nurse tells me Mr Scott is an excellent surgeon, and I feel reassured that everything possible is being done to help me. Poor man – I comment that his work can't be much fun, telling women they have to have their breasts removed. He says that a quarter of his time is spent on surgery and three-quarters on counselling. I decide he does a very good job.

I realize from posters and leaflets that it's European Cancer Week. I certainly chose the right week to learn today's news, I think wryly. At least there should be plenty of information available in the press and on television to help me learn more about this unwelcome intrusion into my life before I make my decision.

Mavis, an old friend who also works with Peter, is waiting for me at reception. Over lunch, several days ago, I had hinted at my problem. Since she lives nearby, she has kindly popped in to see if I need support. We adjourn to the nearest pub and order a large gin and tonic each. As we sit outside in the warm spring sunshine, Mavis's eyes well up as I tell her my news. She admits being too nervous herself to have cancer tests. I talk my thoughts through and decide to keep my problem a secret from all but the boys and my immediate family, my agent and a few trusted friends. In no way must the newspapers get hold of this. I take up Mavis's offer of a lift to Hyde Park from where I can walk to my hairdresser's off Kensington High Street.

Getting out at the park gates I wave Mavis goodbye and head for the Albert Memorial. My head begins to spin and I feel I must sit down. Pigeons flock around the bench in search of titbits, and one in particular catches my eye. Then I realize it isn't a pigeon at all – it's a cockatoo. Beautiful, white and very tame. Someone has lost this lovely bird – I must catch it and take it to the nearest police station. I call to some passers-by to help me. 'Look, it's a cockatoo!' I shout.

They stare back as if I'm mad. The sight of a smartly dressed woman with tears streaming down her face, catching birds in the park, is too much and they move on quickly. I give up and watch the bird rejoin the others, pecking away happily in the gravel.

I can't stay and make a complete spectacle of myself, so I get up and walk quickly on to Ian, my hairdresser and an old friend. As I walk through the door he takes one look, puts his arms around me and hugs me. I can't tell him my secret, but he knows something is terribly wrong. He sits me down and disappears, coming back with a triple brandy which he presses into my hand. He telephones Peter Cranham, my boyfriend, and asks him to come and fetch me.

Without asking any questions he proceeds to do my hair, and once again I bury my face in a magazine. But it's all just a blur.

Peter sees my face as he arrives, and knows it all. Once inside my little flat I sob my heart out. Peter holds me tightly. Of course I realize that life must go on, and being a soggy mess is no help at all. After a while Peter leaves me, more or less together, and I try to do some work. Then I phone Annie Sweetbaum, my agent. She is very upset, but agrees we must cancel some of my work to make time for the operation. If we do this well in advance it will avoid awkward questions from clients who would otherwise feel let down at the last moment.

After that I take a big breath and telephone Tim, my twenty-seven-year-old elder son. I tell him the truth as clearly and unemotionally as I can. He's very sympathetic, and agrees we must meet as soon as possible after my imminent trip to America.

After a quiet supper with Peter I get ready for an early start tomorrow. I have a personal appearance in Maidstone. The show must go on. As I lie in bed, trying to sleep, I wonder what Peter feels. His father recently lost his long painful battle against cancer.

Saturday, 14 May

I wake exhausted. My eyes are red and puffy, and they'll need a good camouflage job on them today.

Nevertheless I arrive in Maidstone in good time to be greeted by the manager of the wonderful new Tudor Park Golf and Sports Centre, who gives me a conducted tour. Soon I'm joined by the other celebrities who will be taking part: Roy Castle, the entertainer, a good friend and workmate, and snooker champion Ray Reardon again. The weightlifter who was to have been with us has had an accident and broken his leg. Sharron Davies, the swimmer, has been taken sick but will try to come along for the evening activities if she's recovered by then. Roy remarks that it's a good job we're both so fit. I smile wryly.

I throw myself into taking two keep-fit sessions, one immediately following the other, and amaze even myself with my brightness and enthusiasm. A quick break for lunch, and then another two energetic sessions followed by autograph signing.

Everyone talks about fitness and healthy living; it makes me feel such a fraud. I wonder if I'll ever do a public exercise session like this again. It's so farcical that I'm being asked for advice when I need help myself. But being a bit of an actress helps at a time like this, so I smile and chatter on.

At supper I find myself sitting next to Roy, who tells me he's on the wagon and comments how good it feels to be fit again, adding: 'But I don't have to tell you that – just look at you.' I quietly comment that things aren't always as they appear. I want to tell him my dreadful secret – but I won't. Why shatter the image? I must keep up the façade, for everyone's sake. I must be positive, and not let myself be pulled down by negative thoughts. From now onwards, each day will be a bonus.

Driving home at midnight, I think ahead to next week and my proposed trip to Florida. I will use the experience and my time in America to strengthen myself both mentally and physically. I'm very fit right now. I've a strong heart and lungs from the nature of my work. My muscles are in tone and I look in good shape. I must keep it this way – strong, and prepared to rid myself of the cancer. I resolve to win the battle.

Sunday, 15 May

Thankfully, a day off. Peter and I tenderly make love, but inwardly I feel so sad and I'm self-conscious about my body.

Nicholas, my younger son of twenty-four, arrives from Bristol early enough to join us for a relaxed breakfast. Peter had phoned him on Friday, hinting that all was not well. It's so good to see him – tall, fine-boned and blond – and he's made such an effort to look nice, which pleases me. Clutching a bunch of flowers, he gives me a knowing hug and a big kiss. Peter tactfully disappears to his office for the morning.

Still sitting in the kitchen, Nic and I settle down to talk. I'm very bright – even amusing – as I tell him my problem. In return he's attentive, enquiring and very understanding. We're honest with one another, but never emotional. It's therapeutic to talk things through with him, someone I can trust, and I can sense his relief on finding me in such good spirits.

Peter returns and suggests lunch out to help us all relax, so we troop off to a favourite Sunday restaurant, Avoirdupois in the King's Road. It's a good lunch with non-stop conversation in an easy, warm atmosphere. A pianist plays our favourite tunes; we laugh, tell jokes and avoid the obvious subject. Nic leaves us late in the afternoon to return to Bristol.

Back at the flat, Peter and I frantically pack for our trip next day and drop into bed exhausted. Unusually for me I take one of the sleeping pills which Mr Scott has prescribed. I don't want any unwanted thoughts keeping me from a good night's sleep tonight.

Monday, 16 May

Going to Florida is a treat Peter has promised me for some time. He goes there frequently on business trips connected with his work as an estate agent, and his American colleagues also come to London quite often. Sometimes they bring their wives, and over the past few years we have become good friends. Working freelance, as I do, creates hectic schedules, which have prevented me from accompanying Peter on previous trips. But come hell or high water, I'm determined to make it this time. Who knows when I'll get the chance again?

Mr Scott agrees it's a good idea, and assures me that as far as he's concerned I have the time. Time, in fact, is on my side, because my cancer has been diagnosed so early.

As we fly off from Heathrow, I notice Peter's spirits are low. I wonder if this is some sort of reaction to the drama of the recent weeks. He quietly hands me a book full of blank pages, and suggests it may help me if I write a daily account of what I'm feeling and going through. It's a kind thought, and, although I feel too lively and ebullient today to do so, I spend some time on the flight writing down what's happened in the last few extraordinary days. That finished, I resolve to have a good time in Florida and not to be a drag on others. Poor Peter has work to do, whereas I, after all, have only play.

Richard Couch, Peter's American business partner, and his wife Sue meet us at Miami Airport. They live and work in America, but are both British. The last time I saw them was in October, when they came to England to be married.

9

Our two-hour car journey to Fort Myers is hot and tiring, but made exciting by a stop in the Everglades to spot alligators. To my amazement, we do. In fact, we see lots of them basking in the murky waters alongside the main road.

Finally we drive on to the mile-long causeway which takes us to Sanibel Island, a beautiful, unspoilt resort on the Gulf of Mexico, a few miles out of Fort Myers. The balcony of our hotel room overlooks miles and miles of exquisite white sandy beaches and beautiful blue sea. I feel I've arrived in paradise.

Tuesday, 17 May

I wake to the sounds of waves crashing on the beach. But pulling back the curtains I'm surprised to find a grey mist instead of sunshine. Can this really be Florida? I thought the sun shone here all the time. Peter tells me it can be dull, but it will still be very hot.

We dress quickly and dash off in our hired car, a white convertible Chrysler le Baron, to Fort Myers. Peter drops me off whilst he goes to his colleague's office for the day. I enjoy getting into the American way of life and quietly amuse myself all day shopping and sight-seeing. Eventually I'm met by the men, who take me with them to visit the land development scheme in which they are both involved some miles outside Fort Myers. It's very interesting, but I secretly wonder if I'll ever come back to see the buildings completed.

Later, back on Sanibel Island, Peter and I make love. But it's difficult to feel abandoned, and afterwards, as I try to sleep, I become apprehensive and wonder just what I'll be like to make love to after the operation.

Wednesday, 18 May

The Florida sun shines today as it should. I make it to the beach. Miles upon miles of white powder. Not sand, but broken shells, ground to a dust by the pounding of the sea. Sanibel is world-famous for its shells, and the beach consists of millions of them, ranging from ordinary to exotic. Collecting shells is the pastime of visitors and inhabitants alike, and all day long the shoreline is littered with people 'bottoms up'. It's infectious, and very soon I become one of them. What a wonderfully therapeutic way to switch off.

Meanwhile Peter has gone about his business, and I have time to myself to reflect on the events of the past month . . . In the *Daily Mail*, some months previously, I had read an article by Teresa Gorman, Conservative MP for Billericay. It was about middle-aged women and the menopause, and how hormone replacement therapy could help overcome some of the problems that women may experience at this time. It also pointed out that if hormone replacement therapy was started soon enough it had another beneficial effect – it strengthened bones and could prevent osteoporosis, a weakening of the bones which affects many women after the menopause and can result in problems such as broken hips, which can lead to complications.

Being a very active woman who wants to keep her mobility – and therefore her independence – into old age, I thought this was worth investigating. A new clinic called the Amarant Centre had just been set up in south London, and I decided to go along. The doctors started out by giving me a thorough medical check-up. I regarded it as a mid-life 'service' and was happy to co-operate with the heart, lung, blood, thyroid, liver and other tests. But I declined the offer of a mammogram – a breast X-ray – since I was already receiving regular check-ups in the West Country. Eventually, however, I conceded and a routine X-ray was taken.

A week later, on 17 April, a message on my answerphone asked me to call the doctor in charge at the Amarant Centre. When I visited him next day he told me there were irregular areas of calcification showing up on my mammogram. I insisted it would be yet another of my familiar lumps, but he shook his head and made an appointment for me to see Mr Scott, a specialist, as soon as possible. I'd gone to the clinic with no problems, but it seemed like I was leaving with a big one.

On the 21st I went along to the Well Woman Clinic held in a large hospital in west London and met Mr Scott. Looking at my X-rays, he confirmed the presence of something other than my usual lumps and requested another mammogram. After having the second mammogram I sat and waited nervously.

'Have I got cancer?' I asked.

Mr Scott looked thoughtful. 'Since you've asked,' he replied, 'I have to tell you that I think you do – but I may be wrong.'

I was stunned and frightened. I had a healthy lifestyle, I ate the right things, I exercised, I didn't smoke. It just didn't add up. Angrily I burst into tears. Mr Scott fetched me a box of tissues and called to his nurse for two coffees.

Then we sat and talked for a long time about my life and work. I explained that I didn't have time to be ill, anyway. I was off to Portugal in two days' time to work at a business convention, keeping everybody fit, and on my return I had to deal with work for books and magazines, for which I had deadlines. Mr Scott was very understanding and arranged to see me again on that fateful Friday, 13 May.

After I had controlled my tears I walked to the car and sat for a long time just looking into space. I decided I would tell no one. Anyhow, it was probably all a mistake . . .

Eventually I arrived home. When Peter opened the door he saw how pale and shaken I looked and enquired anxiously where I had been. As I collapsed into his arms I realized I couldn't keep it to myself. My awful secret had to be shared with somebody.

Now, as I lie soaking up the hot Florida sunshine, thousands of miles away, I think how ironic that this should be happening to me, the presenter of a TV programme entitled *Look Good, Feel Great*.

What a busy schedule I had undertaken over those few weeks. The trip to Albufeira in the Algarve had been hard work but enormous fun. It was for the Stelrad Group, manufacturers of radiators, and along with entertainers Roy Castle and Don

Maclean I had played hostess to the winners of a sales incentive scheme. Hundreds of them flew in from all over England for the week. Don, living in the Midlands, became leader of those flying in from Manchester; Roy to those from Gatwick; and I headed those who had flown in from my home town of Bristol.

The Monte Choro Hotel housed us all, and with its superb sporting facilities enabled the three of us to organize non-stop competitions, fun and games for those who wanted it. And most did. Each morning would start with a keep-fit session in the grounds. After breakfast we had team events in the pool, in the beach club, on the squash courts and on the golf course. The week ended with a gala evening in a local disco, with the three of us doing our bit on stage along with the local cabaret. We had all at some time in our careers worked at Butlin's, and our Redcoat training came in very useful.

When we arrived back in England I had felt tired, but with hardly time to catch my breath had travelled on up to Birmingham to appear live the next morning on *The Time, the Place*. The subject discussed that morning was looks – how important or otherwise they are for success in life.

I take pride in my appearance, but feel it is of less importance than my character. An interesting clash with some young people, including page three models, made me realize that they hadn't yet learnt it to be so. All their hopes and aspirations were hinged on their physical appearance, and I was apprehensive for them in case they found themselves one day stripped of their beauty. It's odd to think how heated I'd felt, but I'm thankful my strict father discouraged vanity and encouraged strength of character when I was a child. I would have been more vulnerable to depression in my present circumstances had I not been so prepared.

My problem was rather more complex than that of the page three girls. My 'good looks' were inextricably intertwined with good health – a healthy body. My livelihood depended on it. If that body seemed somehow less healthy – less perfect, in fact – wouldn't I feel a fraud? Wouldn't other people see me as one? If I had to look in completely new directions for earning my living, I would need all the strength of character my father had encouraged.

In London that afternoon, knowing time was against me, I had urged the publishers to get on with taking the exercise photographs which would be required for the book.

The next day I had travelled back up to Birmingham where, out in the fresh air, we recorded ten pieces of exercise film with members of the Keep Fit Association. A team of women from the Midlands and Avon areas was led by their teacher, Joan, through well-choreographed routines. The women were of mixed age, size and ability, and we hoped it would show the viewer the benefit of simple, well-executed, whole-body movement. Later in the day the crew and I recorded another piece of film from a food exhibition at the National Exhibition Centre in Birmingham. It was on fish, and would be incorporated into the Healthy Living section of the new autumn series of *Look Good, Feel Great.*

It was a long day's work, and so it went on week after week. But being physically busy kept my mind occupied, with little time left to dwell on what I had been told. My problem seemed so incongruous as I threw myself whole-heartedly into work which aimed to make others more aware of their health. A few weeks before, I had flown up to Edinburgh to be guest speaker at the Wits Dinner in aid of St Columba's Hospice. The following morning I was invited to tour the hospice, and stopped to talk to many of those staying there and their families. How unaware I was that day that I too would soon have my own brush with cancer.

Thursday, 19 May

Another lazy day on the beach. After lunch Peter joins me, and we hire bikes to tour the island. Pausing for breath on a little bridge I'm horrified to spot a baby alligator just a few feet away. By the side of the water, it basks in a ray of sunshine glinting through the lush tropical vegetation. We quickly jump back on our bikes and cycle away as Peter remarks that it must have a bigger mum and dad nearby.

The night is balmy. As we drive to meet our friends Sue and Richard we have the roof back and the wind rushes through our hair. All my cares are forgotten as we drink champagne and meet two other English people, Liz and Lawrence, friends of Richard's who are staying in the area for a few days. After a wonderful fish supper at a waterside restaurant, Richard takes us to a bar where we drink, joke and sing into the early morning. Driving back to the hotel I snuggle up to Peter, feeling warm and content.

Friday, 20 May

This is the life for me – it's wonderful, and clothes are no problem in this climate. Just shorts, tee-shirts and flip-flops. We drive into Fort Myers for a typical American breakfast. I order my eggs sunny-side up, and Peter asks for his easy over. It comes with crisp, fine bacon and hash browns, a bit like bubble and squeak. Muffins follow, with a fluffy butter substitute and jam. We wash it all down with endless coffee. Well, that should set us up for the day.

Peter has the day off, and we decide to visit another beautiful hotel with tennis courts, a huge swimming pool and poolside bar. He slips off to get us some drinks and I watch people frolicking and having fun in the water.

Suddenly I find myself ablaze with emotion. I'm obsessed with all the carefree people whose beautiful, healthy bodies surround me, and I fight back tears of jealousy. I feel frightened and alone again, and the tears plop down my bikini-clad chest. I'll never be able to wear a bikini again or lie uninhibited in the sunshine. What a freak I'm going to be.

Peter returns, hands me my drink and understands immediately. He tells me not to worry so much and assures me everything will be all right. But I feel very afraid of the unknown, and threatened by what is going to happen to me. The surgical procedures have all been carefully explained, but I still don't know how I'm going to feel. It's going to be *my* experience, not the doctors'. But the outburst is soon over and I perk up again, forcing myself to take a positive attitude.

Peter buries his head in his book and I lie back enjoying the warm sunshine. My body is relaxed but my mind is busy. So I've got cancer, and I must face the problem as best I can. I *will* get through and conquer it – for my own good, for Peter, for the family and for my friends' sakes. Mentally I'm very determined.

I wonder if there *is* a way of knowing what it will be like. What do you actually feel like after the operation? Does it hurt much? How soon can I get back to normal afterwards? There are so many questions to be answered, and I decide I must find out all I can in the weeks ahead. If I can pre-pare myself with reliable information I know it will go a long way to help my speedy recovery. A bit like preparing for the birth of the children all those years ago. But this time I want facts, not old wives' tales. I need to speak to someone who really knows, someone who's been through it all.

But how can I ask around? I have the same problem as anyone else who appears on television. My private life can become public all too soon. I can just imagine the headlines: 'Fitness Queen Unfit'. Perhaps I could ask amongst my friends and colleagues – people always seem to know someone else who's had cancer. But who can I trust? No, I can't. I'll just have to stay quiet. I'm caught in my own web.

Inside I'm so angry. I feel and look one hundred per cent fit. So why is it happening to *me*?

I had the children when I was young, a lot earlier than most of my friends. And I certainly don't regret that. I think I've been a good mother. But it did mean I wasn't able to pursue my career when I was younger. Now I'm in my prime. I'm at the peak of the career I've so badly wanted and worked so hard for over the years. I've so much more to do, and

I've reached the age when I have the confidence, ability and experience to do it.

I've striven hard so far for my place in society. I've set examples and given my best. I've motivated and helped ordinary people by showing them how to exercise and look after themselves. I'm at a stage in my life when I can be myself, not beholden to others. I have the time and the opportunity to do what I want to do. I love my work on television and radio. I enjoy writing and being able to communicate with ordinary men and women in the street. I don't want to be forced to give it up. I love life.

To have a disease and to die at around fifty wouldn't have been considered so unusual in past generations. But in these health-conscious times most of us in the West have better food, decent housing, good sanitation and plenty of recreation available. Many of the diseases which killed our forefathers are nowadays preventable, and even physical disabilities can largely be overcome by treatment and surgery.

Turning it all over in my mind, I decide it's common sense to take Mr Scott's advice and undergo the surgery. And then, who knows? I may even have another twenty-five healthy years ahead of me to achieve my ambitions. Having made my decision I feel better, and quietly slip into the inviting pool to cool off.

As the afternoon shadows lengthen we return to our hotel, where we pack a bag of beach and party clothes. Jumping into our convertible, we drive off to Fort Myers to join Sue and Richard in the marina. Once aboard their boat, we speed off and head for a tiny private island thirty-five miles away, stopping *en route* to pick up Liz and Lawrence. Richard tells us that this weekend the World Offshore Power Boat Racing Championships are being held locally, and many people will have come from as far away as Miami to see the races.

There are no cars or roads on Useppa Island, and only one little shop. There is, however, a marvellous club house and pool and two small restaurants. As the sun begins to sink on the horizon the only sounds we can hear are the birds, who far outnumber the human inhabitants, and the occasional boat as it purrs past the island.

Saturday, 21 May

After a relaxed breakfast, the men settle down to some paper-work which must be completed over the weekend. I walk to the jetty and watch as the speedboats prepare to move off. I'm appalled to hear the ear-shattering sounds as each twin 500 horsepower engine is started up, and wonder what right man has to ruin the tranquillity of an idyllic dot on a map with such unnecessary noise. I'm glad to see them go, with their brash crews. I find them offensive. Soon Peter and the others arrive, and we climb rather more sedately aboard Richard's boat to join the thousands of other craft far out at sea to watch the race.

Later we arrive at Upper Captiva, yet another enchanting island. As at Useppa, there are no cars here – only a 2000-foot runway which is known to have been used illegally more than once for drug running. At the end of the jetty lies a small, rustic café named after its owner, Barnacle Phil. This grand old character welcomes us with impeccable manners and great charm. Richard tells me Barnacle Phil used to train British World War II fighter pilots in Clearwater, two hours north up the coast near Tampa.

Barnacle Phil's wife is the cook in this basic shed on the beach, where she serves up traditional food to the occupants of passing boats. My cheeseburger is quite definitely the most delicious I have ever tasted. I decide on home-made Key lime pie, a local speciality, to follow, but am soon sharing it out with the others and eating my share of their home-made chocolate cake and pecan pie. Perhaps it's all the fresh air that's making us so appreciative.

We all decide exercise is required, and back on Useppa Island we swim off the excess calories in the club pool. I feel happy and confident, and quietly confirm my determination to win my tussle with cancer. Amazingly, after our feast at Barnacle

Phil's, we find an appetite for supper. Sprucing ourselves up yet again, we spend an elegant evening at the island restaurant.

Sunday, 22 May

This morning I don't feel so good. I have a tickly throat and feel I may be getting a cold. Peter and I enjoy the silence of the island, and during the morning take ourselves off to walk its entire coastline of beautiful sandy beaches.

The birds that have been making so much noise turn out to be ospreys. There are lots of them nesting on tall poles in several parts of the island, and on top of the many wooden channel markers at sea which lead to the island's jetty. What strange birds, to make their enormous nests so uncomfortable and inaccessible. There must be easier places to raise a family.

After a light lunch we swim and laze in the sun. I know I look a picture of health, aglow with fresh sea air and sunshine. And I find it difficult to believe all is not well with my body.

Late in the afternoon we head for home, stopping *en route* at Upper Captiva to savour a pina colada. Back at the hotel I decide on an early night. I must get rid of this sore throat.

Monday, 23 May

Oh dear, we've both got sore throats this morning and feel rough. Peter goes off to work and leaves me to have a quiet day. I wonder if it's the American obsession for air-conditioning that is causing our problem. It's quite intense in many restaurants, hotels and shops, and I've found myself getting very cold indoors having just been very hot outdoors.

The throat feels easier as the day goes on, and Peter and I join Mark Alexander, another business colleague, his family and friends at home in Fort Myers for supper. It's interesting to see Americans entertaining at home. They really are most hospitable.

Tuesday, 24 May

The weather's not so hot today, so we decide to go to town and shop. Rayban sunglasses for Nic. Colourful sweatshirts for Tim and Peter's daughter Holly. A jog suit and Reeboks for Peter. Socks for me. We decide we've been eating too much, so go without lunch. After sight-seeing we return to the hotel and relax in the gardens, reading our books.

Later, in the evening, we drive to a nearby hotel on the beach which has a disco. As arranged, we meet up with Richard and Sue and some other friends. I've put on a smart black and white two-piece – more suited to London, I decide, as I watch the girls arrive. My tan is covered up by long sleeves and a shirt neckline, whereas they are looking wonderful in low-cut dresses with bare arms.

Suddenly I feel out of place and insecure. Everyone else chatters happily, but I don't feel part of it. I feel different. I've got cancer. They have everything to look forward to in their lives. But what do I have? What's my future? I just don't know.

As the girls become more flirty and fun I become more withdrawn. I feel desperate. I feel envious of everyone. I feel so old, a has-been. I try to put on a brave face and make small talk, but as Peter dances with me and holds me tight I close my eyes and bury my head in his shoulder. I feel a failure, and soon I'm going to be ugly.

I try to stifle my crying, and look up to see Richard and Sue watching me. Richard dances closer and knowingly squeezes my arm. I realize he's in on my secret. Peter must have told him. He said he might.

I feel claustrophobic. We politely excuse ourselves. I say that I'm overtired and my throat is sore, and we quickly leave. I realize I've lost my self-control and I've let my feelings get the better of me. I'm so ashamed of myself and sorry for Peter. In front of his colleagues I've let him down. I've acted like a spoilt child. My father wouldn't have approved.

We drive the short distance to our hotel in silence, but Peter has his hand tightly on mine. I can't get into the safety of our room quickly enough. I feel so incredibly angry. I hate myself. I hate cancer. I hate everything. I hate everybody.

I loosen my shoes and kick them across the room. I throw my clothes off in a rage and hit out at Peter, who tries to comfort me. Blazing with hate and jealousy and totally out of control I shout: 'Why me? Why me? What have I done to deserve this?' I throw myself on to the bed in despair, and drown in a sea of self-pity.

Peter tries to talk to me gently, but knows I can't be reasoned with. Sleep is the only answer, and he quickly reaches for the pills Mr Scott prescribed for me ('In case you find the need,' he said). He must have known from his experience that one day the dreadful moment of realization would finally hit me in this way.

Wednesday, 25 May

Peter is very quiet this morning and looks sad as he leaves for the office. Sue phones and invites me to spend the day at home with her. I arrive red-eyed and sheepish. I feel guilty about last night's outburst, but she is incredibly kind and understanding as I tumble out my problems. I feel cross, tired and confused. She listens quietly. In her mid-thirties, she is a handsome, strong, open-natured girl as tall as myself, which I find strangely comforting this morning. I feel at ease with her.

I'd liked her natural, unaffected manner from the start when Richard introduced us to her in London early last year. After a whirlwind courtship they were married in the autumn. Peter and I just managed to get to the wedding reception in Worcestershire by flying to Birmingham Airport from Crete, where I had been invited to help publicize tourism.

Now, here in Florida, I find she too is having problems. She's trying to cope with the difficult task of adjusting from her outdoor life of horse breeding and training, in the English countryside, to the American way of life in a high-rise town apartment. One of her horses, Celtic Shot, was a winner at this year's Cheltenham Festival races. It can't have been easy for her, leaving all that behind for others to run. As Sue and I talk, we decide we can both help ourselves through our difficult, although very different, times by being cheerful and positive. We must not be miserable or moan. We conclude our task over the next few months is to surrender our independence temporarily and give full support to our men, who in turn will provide us with the love and strength we need to adjust to our new situations.

I relax. At last I've found an ally. One I can trust. When the men apprehensively return home, they can see our cheerfulness and decide, perhaps with relief, to open a bottle of champagne to celebrate. We toast all our futures, which suddenly look brighter.

Thursday, 26 May

Sadly, this is our final day in America. We lie back and soak up the sun for the last time. I feel optimistic, and decide I will return to Florida and this little piece of heaven one day.

We hire bikes and spend several hours cycling to the lighthouse at the end of the island. After lunch we walk for miles along the white beach, joining the shell-seekers. Later we visit Periwinkle Gardens, an area of small, select boutiques and shops clustered around a cool, leafy wood. Peter buys me a stunning turquoise and pink tracksuit as an early birthday present – it will be pretty and practical to wear after my operation. We also buy some champagne and plastic disposable champagne flutes for a small thank you party we'll throw tonight.

The gathering is fun. Our guests are noisy and extrovert – no doubt encouraged by the bubbly. We all move off in due course to the hotel restaurant nearby, where we have reserved a very large table. Conversation and laughter are ceaseless, only halted by the dramatic entrance of the chef bearing what looks like a birthday cake. To my embarrassment he sidles up to me and proceeds to give a little speech, saying how all our American friends and colleagues have enjoyed our visit. He places the cake in front of me and I blow out the candles. It's bright green, and not a cake at all but a huge, delicious Key lime pie. 'Good Luck Green Goddess' is written across the top.

I'm taken aback and very touched. What a lovely surprise. With moist eyes I stand up and mumble my thank yous. Peter smiles. What a memorable trip this has been, and how warm these people are.

Friday, 27 May

Not surprisingly, I've got a bit of a headache this morning. I pack for our return journey later this afternoon and carefully place our precious shell collection between clothes for safety.

At the air terminal we wait for an internal flight to Miami. Black clouds are gathering, however, and a storm is brewing. We climb into the small aircraft, which holds about ten people, and strap ourselves into the basic seats. The person who we think is our hostess, smart in her uniform, turns out to be the captain of the aircraft and she welcomes us aboard. She warns us it may well be a bumpy, uncomfortable flight, and suggests we keep our seat belts fastened.

After take-off we laugh and joke nervously as she fights to duck and dive the storm whirling around us. I'm not a bad traveller and am rarely nervous, but this time I admit to myself I'm scared. I glance apprehensively at Peter and hold his hand tightly. The atmosphere is very hot and sweaty in the cramped plane, and I can feel the tension mounting. I try to relax, but the grisly thought occurs to me that perhaps this is the way I'll snuff it. Rather dramatic, I think, but at least together with Peter.

Somewhat later than scheduled we land safely at Miami, where it's raining torrentially. We look out over the city, dark, wet and thunderous, and laugh – somewhat with relief – to see all the ground crew wearing yellow oilies including sou'westers. It reminds us both of our fishermen friends in Dorset. So much for fabulous Florida – it looks more like winter in England!

Saturday, 28 May

Maggie, my cat, is delighted to see us when we pick her up from the cattery in Weybridge, suitably called 'A Country Hotel for Cats'. She has been very well looked after, as usual, by Jean.

Maggie, a dainty little tabby with perfect markings, was part of a litter that Ian, my hairdresser, found himself with several years ago. Knowing I missed Poppy, my jet-black cat which I left in Bristol with my ex-husband, he suggested I look at a black and white in his litter. But my eye was caught by a fluffy tabby bundle which cocked its head eagerly on one side as if to say: 'Please have me.' The black and white one didn't stand a chance. I took the tabby home, intending to call her Tiger, but Peter immediately called her Margaret – after our leader, he laughingly said. Less than one year later Maggie produced four beautiful kittens, all just like herself with their stripy markings. How I would love to have kept them all.

Soon, back in the flat, I'm stuck into the household chores. Peter has driven into his West End office to make sure they have coped in his absence. They have.

Sleep comes soon. We've lost five hours. But there's not much rest for the wicked, and I have to do my bit for Telethon '88, the mammoth fund-raising event taking place all over Britain this holiday weekend.

Sunday, 29 May

Up at 7 a.m., and soon we're on the road heading north to Castle Donnington, where I'm to appear for Central TV at a big keep-fit event called Shape '88. It's being staged by a company who run lots of fitness centres in the Midlands, and the proceeds of the day will go towards Telethon '88, much of which is organized and televised by the ITV companies.

For many years I have helped the BBC with their Children in

Need appeal, acting as one of their presenters from the BBC's West Country studio, so I'm used to the energy and enthusiasm these occasions generate. The atmosphere this morning is electric as I arrive at the sports centre. Pop music pulsates, and men and women of all shapes and ages gyrate and contort as they follow their leaders through exercise-to-music sessions. I quickly change into my tights and sweatshirt, emblazoned with the logo of Central TV's health and fitness programme *Look Good, Feel Great*, which I co-present.

Soon it's my turn to be teacher, and for an hour my large class twist and turn. Everyone is happy as we bend and stretch, many of them for the third or fourth time today. It's amazing how exercising can give one energy rather than sap it, when one is doing it at a steady pace and listening to one's own body for signs of exhaustion. The session over, I shower, change and cool off. Then I sign autographs and talk to the crowd.

In the afternoon, as the event begins to wind down, we leave the leisure centre and get back on the road to drive to Birmingham. Events are already taking place and being transmitted live from the large halls of the National Exhibition Centre, which is the nerve centre for Central's contribution to Telethon '88. The whole area is a buzz of activity. But I'm tired, and after an early supper crash into bed because, once again, I've an early start in the morning.

Monday, 30 May

Bank holiday for some, but not for me. Up at 5.45, I shower, wash my hair and change into my green *Look Good, Feel Great* tracksuit. With a surprising spring in my step I walk to the huge hall of the Exhibition Centre, leaving Peter sleeping soundly. Jet lag seems to have caught up with him today. My own throat is very sore, and my husky voice is going to be a big problem this morning. I feel awful really. I'm very hot and I think I've got a temperature. But I act bright and lively. After all, I'm the keep-fit lady and this is what's expected of me.

The place is jumping. Schoolchildren, boy scouts and celebrities are everywhere. Gary Terzza, presenter for children's ITV, is the compere this morning. He and almost everyone else in the hall have been working throughout the night and still have hours more to go.

I feel mischievous as I eye my pupils for the keep-fit session, which I will perform live at about eight o'clock. Dressed in yellow are about three hundred Telecom telephonists, constantly taking calls and donations from the public. They can be my guinea pigs. A few minutes before I get the signal to jump into action, the relief telephonists arrive and file into the studio. They're good sports and say they too will take part. The children need no encouragement, and as we go live everyone joins in the fun. It's hectic. With phones in one hand the telephonists twist and stretch as best they can while we do exercises for the neck, chest and arms. When the rest of us start jumping, they, still seated, stamp their feet. All in all we chaotically enjoy ourselves, and must make an amusing and colourful spectacle for the viewers at home to chuckle over their cornflakes at.

Soon it's over and we collapse laughing. I only hope some of the tensions and strains of working all night in the hall will have been relieved. But, more optimistically, I hope some viewers may be persuaded to take a little exercise themselves and dig into their pockets to improve our financial figures for Telethon '88. Later I discover that Central TV raised £3 million.

I return to the hotel and, after checking out, drive on to Sutton Park where I meet up with other entertainers and personalities on Central's roadshow and join in the big, day-long celebrations. By now, I'm quite hoarse.

When we arrive back home, late in the afternoon, Peter puts on the answerphone to listen to messages. He's angry and I'm upset as we hear Jan Leeming's pretty voice expressing her concern on hearing I have been unwell. Apparently Mavis, out of her concern for me, had foolishly told a mutual friend my news. I go hot and cold and wonder who else knows by now. I must put an end to this or my secret will be out before I've even had my treatment. I've work to do until then to pay the bills, and I can't afford to have people idly chattering about me, however well intentioned. My throat hurts a lot, I've lost my voice and I feel very low. Bed is the only answer.

Tuesday, 31 May

Thank goodness I've got a day off. At last I've time to catch my breath. As I do the ironing I begin to wonder when my treatment will begin, if I confirm that I will be going ahead with it. Apprehensively, I ring Mr Scott's secretary to find out. But she tells me no decision has been made. However, she gives me an appointment to see Mr Crosswell, the reconstructive surgeon, on 8 June.

I feel depressed and begin to question whether I want treatment, let alone an operation. Should I just ignore it all, and let nature take its course? Perhaps the cancer will go away. I've often heard people talk about alternative cures, and I've recently read about people helping themselves by diet and positive thinking. Should I take the chance? Others seem to have had success – why not me? I remain deep in thought for the rest of the day.

Later I pick up the phone and speak to Jan Leeming. I tell her I have not been unwell, but hint that I may have a problem. She's a little embarrassed, and then tells me of a concert she recently compered. After the show she spoke to the talented singer who was the star of the evening, and said she was puzzled as to why she hadn't seen much of her recently on television. The girl told Jan she had been ill, but because of the publicity clients were put off and her work had suffered. Now that's exactly what could happen to me. Jan understands and wishes me well. Mavis sounds mortified as I phone to tell her the news has spread.

JUNE

Wednesday, 1 June

A new month – rabbits! I've a dental check-up this morning. Fortunately my teeth aren't often a problem. However, this time the dentist asks me to make a further appointment in the next few weeks as he needs to do some work on an old filling. I'm hesitant about dates, explaining that I'm due to go into hospital soon for surgery but don't know exactly when. He politely enquires why, just for his records. Reluctantly, I tell him I may have cancer.

He lights up with enthusiasm and yet concern as he confides that he, too, had cancer twenty years ago. I look at this fine, strong figure of a man and take heart. He says if I have the opportunity for surgery I must take it and be positive in my attitude. *He* did, and with great success. He wishes me luck and gives me an early appointment for the next week.

I arrive at my agent's busy office and am greeted by Annie herself and her 'angels', as she calls her staff. We talk over the work I have in hand and what I won't be able to do. It's been widely reported in the press recently that I will be taking the new exercise-to-music course which I have helped the Sports Council and the Royal Society of Arts to launch. I've blocked out three or so weeks to enable me to do this comprehensive new course, and I know it will take up a lot of my energy and brainpower. But it will set a good example to other keep-fit teachers, especially the new young ones, and help clear up the muddle about how to teach exercise classes to music correctly and safely. I have been looking forward to the challenge, and with my usual thirst for knowledge I was determined to be one of the first (hopefully) to pass the exam. However, Annie and I decide it's not to be.

The pantomime is my biggest disappointment of all. Playing Fairy Godmother at Hastings last Christmas was so much fun, and to be offered the part again this Christmas in a theatre a little nearer home, at Bognor Regis, was really good news. But what state am I going to be in after the operation? What will I look like and how will I feel? Will I have the energy for all the travel and demands of pantomime? I have become increasingly apprehensive and nervous over the past few weeks – especially at the thought of letting down the cast and public at the last minute. I decide to pull out. Doing so now shouldn't cause too much concern for the management, who have time to recast. So, with my future uncertain, I grudgingly admit defeat and Annie cancels me out.

Back at the flat I open my post. A letter from John, my ex-husband, is very touching. We were married for twenty-five years and remain good friends. Well aware of my history of breast lumps, he is disturbed and concerned to have learnt from Nic that I am to have another spell in hospital. He writes that nature has been very kind to me in many ways, but 'does appear to turn a little spiteful from time to time', and that he would have thought I'd had my fair share of the surgeon's knife. He adds that he is saddened to learn of my news, and anxious for me, but knows that with my grit and determination I will bounce back with even more energy. On a lighter note he comments that Nic had told him I was to have a vasectomy! I disappear into the bathroom and have a good cry.

Thursday, 2 June

Today I'm having lunch with Jill Passmore, originally a workmate from my fashion days but now a close friend. A Cornishwoman full of common sense, she has a keen sense of humour which keeps her sane in her high-powered public relations job in the textile and fashion world. She's always cheerful, and over many years we have helped and encouraged each other through various ups and downs.

We met in connection with the Devon County Show in Exeter, where for six years I ran and produced the Show theatre. For four days in May a year's organization came to fruition. Every year I was anxious as I watched the first two-and-a-half-hour performance live on stage. But I was always calmed by the words of the Show boss, John Hockin, an old soldier, who would remind me that if my preparations had been thorough I could expect good results. I would also apply one of my mother's sayings about housework – that if you look after the corners the middle will look after itself. There must have been some truth in this, for every year the theatre turned out to be a huge success.

It was a job I was reluctant to give up when I joined the BBC for Breakfast Time, but it was too much to continue with. I auditioned the acts as well as organizing the stage, the seating, the scenery, the lighting and the sound equipment. And I remember the paperwork involved, the timing, the running orders, the publicity, and arranging the back-stage changing facilities and the front-of-house cleaning up. And all those rehearsals. Finally the non-stop performances three times daily, which I helped to compere. I wonder how on earth I did it all, and recall the biggest nightmare of all – finance. For months before the Show I would seek sponsorship. Sometimes, if I was lucky, it came from a single company. But often it was from several companies collectively.

We produced a wonderful variety of live entertainment. The centrepiece was a truly first-class fashion show – I used all my contacts to put together every year a show worthy of anything that London could offer. The accompanying entertainment would be international in flavour – we had Spanish dancers, musicians from South America, the band of the Royal Marines, top-flight electronic organists, and much more besides.

The one essential link every year, just in case it should all get a little too international and metropolitan and citified for the West Country folk, was a fantastic entertainer known as the Wag from Widecombe. Tony Beard was a genuine Devon farmer and a very colourful character. He always had me and the audience in stitches as he performed his comedy routines in true yokel style, the soft West Country burr filtered through the straw in his mouth.

There were so many amusing moments in that theatre. Like the time I got tongue-tied on stage introducing the Pheasant Pluckers from Plymouth! Or when I needed to thank a local dignitary for the loan of her riding accessories which added authenticity to a country-style fashion show. Obviously nervous, I thanked her for her hunting hot and crap instead of her hat and crop.

But by far the most embarrassing moment was caused by a knitted wedding dress made from the finest wool. It didn't arrive in time for the start of the spectacular fashion show being performed before the County Show committee, guests and press. The final scene was set and Kim, the beautiful bride, appeared. Everyone gasped. The designer had omitted the necessary petticoat and the dress was see-through. Kim was, indeed, a blushing bride. The following day the Star carried her picture and the story – not quite the right image for a County Show!

One of my nicest tasks each year was to receive the royal guest in the theatre and introduce him or her to the cast. Prince Charles was the most interested of all the royals I had the privilege of escorting, and was extremely amusing company.

And it was in one of those years that I met Jill, who at that time promoted British Wool. I went to another County Show, in Malvern, Worcestershire, to meet her and see a fashion show she had produced. We hit it off instantly and I recall ducking and diving to avoid the torrential rain (usual Show weather) as we ran to her hospitality stand to talk. There we agreed our business, then settled down to the equally important business of celebrating our deal with a glass or two of wine. She would help sponsor my show in Devon, and we continued to do convivial *business over the years. Later, I was to be photographed in her British Wool fashions and presented her trade videos for worldwide exposure.*

Today's lunch begins in our usual cheerful, noisy way. We chatter about business. Hers is International Linen nowadays, not British Wool. As usual in the fashion trade she talks of several seasons in advance, and as she does so I become painfully aware of my uncertain future. Will I wear the colours and shapes she describes?

I begin to feel distant from Jill, who, sensing my discomfort, asks me what I'm up to these days. I decide to tell her my secret. She's optimistic, and reminds me of a time seven or eight years ago when we lunched together the day before I went into hospital with a previous lump in my breast. It had been surgically removed, and I was fit and back in action in no time at all. She remarks how well I look today, and in her wise, old-fashioned Cornish way says she knows I'll be all right because my coat looks glossy and my hair and eyes are bright. I hope she's right.

In the early evening Peter joins me at a small reception to launch a young interior designer friend of ours in Battersea. Stephanie bubbles her way through a good crowd of friends and business acquaintances as we drink champagne and toast her success in her new shop. Her father, Chris, a distinguished Admiral's Cup sailor, and her mother, Audrey, good friends of ours, are there to support her. The shop is very prettily decorated. Could it be that (it's my colour, green) or maybe the champagne that's making me feel happy and more relaxed this evening?

Afterwards we make our way over Albert Bridge to the new and prestigious Chelsea Harbour development. From my Battersea flat I've watched it grow. Those in Chelsea would say I'm the wrong side of the river, but I love being there.

Tonight Lord Linley, Princess Margaret's son, is giving a large reception to celebrate the opening of his new restaurant, Deals, which is in the middle of the complex. The courtyard outside the restaurant, roofed by a huge glass dome, is packed tight with hundreds of people. The press stalk the slight Lord Linley and his leggy on/off girlfriend, Susannah Constantine. Familiar faces from television, stage and society columns abound, and as we walk through the door my old friend and workmate Glynn Christian, the cook from BBC *Breakfast Time*, comes up and gives me a kiss. We stay together sipping champagne, but finally decide it's time to eat.

Peter drives us to Pucci's pizza restaurant, a favourite of ours in the King's Road, where we reminisce and laugh about our many escapades together during our mornings on *Breakfast Time*. Tonight all my cares are forgotten.

Friday, 3 June

I finish writing my contribution to the book *Look Good, Feel Great*, which will be published in September to tie in with the TV series. As I send off my copy I can only hope that I too will be looking good and feeling great at the book's launch. I pack some casual clothes, put Maggie in her wire travelling basket, and drive off to Dorset for the weekend.

Peter's small house, overlooking the harbour at Mudeford, near Christchurch, feels warm and welcoming as I open the front door. I let Maggie out of her cage and quickly put down water, food and a tray of cat litter. She heads straight for her tray and obligingly performs. I take stock of the food cupboards and fridge and pop out to the local shops for supplies. Then I cook myself a light supper which I take upstairs to the lounge.

The view from here is splendid. Tonight colourful boats are bobbing up and down on the calm waters. People amble past the window and on down to the quay with its quaint cottages, fishing boats and lobster pots. They walk the paths along the harbour and over the open grassland where children and dogs play happily. Maggie settles on my lap as I savour the delights of the sunset, and only moves when she hears Peter's key in the lock. Soon she is settled on *his* lap. The three of us are quiet and content.

Saturday, 4 June

After a good night's sleep I'm up early, preparing myself for a photographic session. Although Mudeford is our place of rest, I've work to do today. I've written an article for the Rolls Royce Enthusiasts' Club magazine, and it's going to be illustrated with a series of exercise photographs. We'll be shooting them alongside an old Rolls Royce, parked deep in the New Forest. I've arranged to work over this weekend as I'm anxious to complete the job whilst I'm still able to.

At the agreed place we meet up with the editor. Malcolm is an enthusiast and is producing the magazine, called *Pinnacle*, as a labour of love. He's driven down from Bath this morning in a magnificent 1920 yellow, beige and brown Rolls Royce. It's in beautiful condition, complete with all interior extras including the original silver scent bottles and spirit flasks. In fact, all one might need for a day out in the country!

On the way Malcolm has picked up Jeremy and his wife Jinx in Andover. Jeremy is a keen amateur photographer, and Jinx his assistant for the day. With their other hats on he is a dentist and she an air hostess.

We work hard throughout the morning, but fast-moving clouds affect the lighting and make continuity a problem. At 1.30 we finish, just as it begins to rain – good timing. We adjourn to the nearest Forest pub. As we say goodbye, I secretly hope the films are processed very soon so I can have the selected shots in time to caption them.

Peter's mother lives in the area, and I feel she should know what's going on – Peter may need her help. We call at her house and talk to her over tea. She's not one to show her feelings readily, but we can see she's devastated for us, and fully understands the strain we're both under. But I'm determined not to show any signs of a problem as we join our local friends later for a night out in Lymington. Everyone says how well Peter and I look from our trip to Florida.

Back in the house I realize it's been a long day. I don't think I shall need much rocking tonight.

Sunday, 5 June

A bit hung over, we busy ourselves with domestic chores – while Peter washes the car I get on with the gardening. It's only a small plot, but we have window boxes and tubs as well. I pop out to the local garden centre to buy geraniums and pansies to add colour, together with some shrubs. After I plant them it looks good, and I hope it will continue to flower decoratively till I can tend it again, later in the summer.

We both love walking, and every weekend that we're down here we take ourselves off to plod along the local beach or over the headland or into the Forest. Today, as we walk alongside the harbour, Peter spies David, a close friend and one of last night's crowd in the restaurant in Lymington. David is the boss of a big motor dealership in Bournemouth but also a keen amateur fisherman. He shows us a new motorboat he's bought to go sea fishing in. It's American, a Bayliner, and David shows it off like a little boy with a new toy. It's a bit flashy for Mudeford but it certainly looks the business. Peter and I had inspected the Bayliner range of small boats in the showroom and marina in America, where they're very popular. I can see Peter's a bit envious – he has a small dinghy of his own which he keeps in the garage, but we haven't had time to put it in the water this year. I feel a tinge of sadness for him as I wonder how much boating he'll do this summer. What a killjoy I'm going to be.

Monday, 6 June

Up early for Peter to catch the six o'clock train back to London. As I clear up the house I feel weary and still annoyed that I may have become the subject of social chit-chat. I don't want everybody to know my horrid secret – I just want a few close friends and my family to support me. I certainly don't want to be reminded about my problems by nosey parkers and know-it-alls wherever I go.

I make myself a coffee and look at the books and leaflets Mavis gave me about the Bristol Cancer Self Help Centre, for which she raises funds. In the car on my journey back to London, I play their tape 'Living with Cancer'. I begin to feel depressed and confused, and for some reason feel guilty about contemplating surgery. Every time I think about it I feel I'm letting down the keep-fit profession. I start to wonder again if there's an alternative treatment for me.

Back in the flat, Peter seems low. Perhaps he's worried about business, but I think he's more concerned about me. The phone rings and a smile comes back on my face. Nic's going to visit us in Mudeford next weekend. Good.

Tuesday, 7 June

This morning I work on plans to write four quarterly articles about keeping fit for a Ford Motor Company house magazine, *Front Desk*. They're to be accompanied by relevant photographs. Gary, whose project it is, has come to discuss the details and suggests the first article could appear in August. I panic and persuade him that November would be better. Even then, the copy will need to be in by late September. He's quite happy with my suggestion and I'm relieved. It should give me time to convalesce and get back into shape for the photographs.

Late in the afternoon, I ring Tim at home in Dartmouth. To my surprise John, his father, is visiting him and so we have a short chat. He's very kind. I want Tim to visit me, and suggest he might come either to London or Mudeford soon. But he seems to be too busy, what with teaching at the Naval College and all his other tasks. He says he's sorry, but he'll see what he can do in a few weeks' time.

As I put down the phone, I feel a sense of rejection. Surely Tim could fit me into his tight schedule somewhere if he wanted to? I need to see him. I know I'm his mother, to whom he can come when he's in trouble – but damn it, *I'm* in trouble now and I need his support badly. Maybe he just can't cope with the idea that his mother has cancer – but I still feel choked.

There's a programme about cancer on the television, which makes Peter and me feel despondent. I hate this blasted cancer. It's taking over our lives. We talk about how we're going to tackle it. Will I be told I need radiotherapy and chemotherapy? Why don't I forget about it for the time being and see what I'm like in six months' time? Should I ignore it completely, and let nature take its course? Who knows, it may go away. I've been through all this in my mind before, and got nowhere. Tomorrow I'm seeing the reconstructive surgeon, Mr Crosswell. Will he be able to help, or will he merely add to my doubts and fears? My head is full of muddles as I tearfully try to sleep.

Wednesday, 8 June

Time for another haircut. Nearly a month since that terrible Friday the 13th when I last saw Ian, but I don't seem much further on and I've nothing positive to show for my month's anguish.

Back in the flat, I find my family and friends are beginning to rally round me. David, my ex-brother-in-law in Australia, has written to me having heard the news, and my cousin Mary from Somerset has also sent a letter. She has her hands full already. In her forties, she's expecting her fourth baby in the autumn. Her first little girl is still only four. Ironically, Mary's a midwife. It's comforting to hear from them both. To my surprise, my next envelope contains an early birthday card from my brother in the West Country. Anthony has heard from the boys that I'm ill, and wants to know where and when I'm going into hospital. It's the first contact I've had with him in five years, since my separation from John and my leaving the West Country. Can this be the credit side of having cancer, that it reunites brothers and sisters? I write back giving him details.

Central TV's *Something to Treasure* is on this afternoon. I watch nervously because I am today's guest, talking about my collection of pictures. I paint still life and landscape in oils when I have the time – which isn't often nowadays. I begin by showing one of my own flower paintings, but it pales into insignificance beside a still life I own by my old friend George Bruce, the eminent portrait painter. His small still lifes and landscapes are as impressive as his huge commissioned portraits. I was a sitter for him some years ago, and over my frequent visits watched him paint this particular still life.

The pictures I collect are not usually expensive – just those which catch my eye. The last one shown on the programme, a watercolour I bought recently, is by local Christchurch artist Christopher Hollick. It's an interesting picture, not least because it shows the view from our lounge window in Mudeford. A pretty sailing boat, depicted in the foreground in the marshy beds at the edge of the harbour, lies where it finally came to rest, having broken free from its mooring during the hurricane of October last year. The programme comes over well and I'm pleased with the result.

I feel a need to put my house in order. I look through my accounts and find some outstanding monies owed to me. I send the individuals concerned a reminder, although I find it annoying to have to chase people up. I call my accountant, who I find is himself unwell, but ask his assistant to complete my accounts for the past year. I ring my solicitor to have him finalize my divorce settlement. My will is in order. As I finish my tasks, my air of efficiency fades and I feel very scared, vulnerable, tired and alone.

Late in the afternoon a taxi takes me to Mr Crosswell's consulting rooms. I'm shown into the comfortable waiting room, where I sit with my nose in a magazine. I hear a door close and look up, and see in the reception area the back of a gentleman who reminds me of Mr Scott. Almost immediately I'm called, and as I enter Mr Crosswell's room I'm greeted by Mr Scott, whom I had not expected to see.

Mr Crosswell talks quietly to me, and about me to Mr Scott as I'm shown into an ante-room for examination. I sit on the side of the couch as both men come in to take a look at me. Mr Crosswell takes a Polaroid picture of my chest. They retreat into the consulting room and I quickly dress. Mr Crosswell has a quizzical look on his face, but can't give me a decision on whether, let alone how, he can operate. He feels he must give it more thought, and asks me to come back on Friday morning. I feel it's all a bit woolly and vague – something of an anti-climax.

Mr Scott gives me a lift back to Mayfair, where I can catch a ride home with Peter from the office. The distance is short, but the journey takes a long time because of the rush hour traffic. However, it gives me the opportunity to fire questions at poor Mr Scott who, as before, answers them carefully and thoroughly. In answer to my first anxious question he tells me I won't need radiotherapy or chemotherapy, which are not necessary after an operation for non-invasive cancer. I'm greatly relieved, not least because, with this follow-up treatment and its side-effects, I would have been unable to work for a very long time. I then want to know what effect the op. will have on my muscles. Will I be able to exercise again, and how long will I be out of action?

I'm so pleased to see him today. He is officially on holiday, and I feel reassured that I'm getting the best possible help. He tells me to love and support Peter now, because Peter will need to be strong to give me strength later, when *I'll* need it.

Over supper, at the Brasserie in the Fulham Road, Peter and I talk and make plans. At last, in bed, he tenderly makes love to me, but though I want to I can't respond. I just cling very close to him and cry my heart out. We both feel very sad tonight.

Thursday, 9 June

Back with the dentist this morning. He gives me a small injection in my arm and I relax back as he removes an old filling and replaces it.

I'm still a bit dopey from the drugs, so I hail a cab to the West End model agency whose books I'm on for the occasional TV commercial or photographic assignment. Richard Patching, my producer from *Look Good, Feel Great*, and his secretary are already there with Tom and Cheryl, the agency bosses. Together we go through the hundreds of photographs sent in by teenagers, potential models, in response to a competition the agency and programme are running jointly. It's a difficult task, but eventually we select the finalists. The finals themselves will be filmed in July, and I secretly know I won't be there on that occasion. It's one I shall be sorry to miss.

Suzanne, my producer's secretary, has brought the photographs from the session I did at the Peak Fitness Club at the Hyatt Carlton Hotel in London. They will appear in the book that ties in with the programme. I settle down and put them in sequence, selecting the best shots which show the correct positioning for the exercises. I have to concentrate hard. I can't afford to make a mistake at this stage.

It's Thursday late-night shopping in Oxford Street, and unusually I have an hour or two to myself. I think I'll go to Selfridge's. In the underwear department I gaze at the satins and silks, the frills and lace, and decide to spoil myself. I'll buy myself something pretty, something to boost my morale. I try on a white teddy, a lacy all-in-one. Yes, this can be the inspiration I need, a spur to help me get myself back into shape after the operation.

I'm pleased with my present to myself and put it away carefully in a drawer to keep it safe for a later date. I'm more content this evening. Peter and I make love and settle down to a good night's sleep.

Friday, 10 June

Mr Crosswell sees me immediately I arrive. He has had time to consider how he may be able to reconstruct my breasts after the operation. He draws diagrams, and shows me where the incisions may be made for Mr Scott to rid me of the cancer and for him to insert a prosthesis. But it isn't straightforward and will depend on the elasticity of my skin, my circulation, the extent of breast tissue removed and the damage incurred.

He explains how he may insert a temporary prosthesis, which would gradually be inflated in the days and weeks after the operation. It would slowly and comfortably expand with my skin, and would eventually be removed and replaced by a permanent prosthesis, a bag of silicone gel, in an operation at a later date.

Because of the nature of my work – physical exercise with lots of movement – he feels the prosthesis would best be put directly under my skin and not covered by muscle. Usually muscle is brought around from the back and flapped over the prosthesis, thus protecting it. In my case, however, the prosthesis might be displaced and move to one side as I exercise. Oh dear, it all sounds so awful.

He smiles and tells me that this would not be a disaster but might be embarrassing. I'm worried about the prosthesis being rejected, but he assures me this is most unlikely. He says at least one of my nipples and the areola are likely to be removed during the operation. I'm horrified. But he goes on to explain how even these can be remade from my own skin, taken from areas of darker skin, such as the groin, for the areola, and from somewhere like the lobe of the ear for the nipple.

He makes it all sound so simple, and I begin to feel it's not going to be quite so bad after all. I suppose it's normal and everyday to him. I relax and we joke with one another, which makes it easier.

For about three months I'll have to wear a sort of corset all the time to support me and keep everything in place. The 'nipple making' would be yet another operation in the months to come. However, he says, if I require these for cosmetic reasons, stick-on versions are available. We both chuckle.

I ask him whether I'll ever be able to wear a bikini again, and he assures me I will. I laugh as I tell him that I can't see myself going topless again in the future. Maybe I'll have to wear this year's beach fashion of a beautiful flower stuck over where my nipples should be instead. I don't know whether to laugh or cry. What I'm hearing is all so amazing and such a shock – though a pleasant one.

Mr Crosswell tells me I'm lucky. That word again. This time I'm lucky because I have small boobs, and that means fewer cuts. But it also means that, had I wanted to replace my slight figure with big boobs, it would have caused problems for my skin and circulation. What a shame to miss such an opportunity!

What problems and laughter my small breasts had caused me over the years. What teasing I had during puberty from my brother, his friends and the boys at my co-ed grammar school in Bristol. What panic I'd had each time I found a lump during the past twenty years.

I was so shy that I couldn't tell my mother I wanted a bra like everyone else at school, so I went out and bought myself one secretly. I washed it every night and dried it under the eiderdown so that she wouldn't find it. I so desperately wanted to be like the other well-developed girls.

Remarkably, when it came to breast-feeding I managed rather well. So much so that, because I produced so much milk, I had to wear those horrid little glass things over my nipples and supplied the milk bank with the excess milk my small breasts couldn't contain.

As a model, my two fried eggs became a bit of a joke. Although, looking round back-stage, not too many of my friends had much to boast about either. And at the start of BBC's Breakfast Time *I recall my embarrassment when the newspapers reported I had the ideal figure and well and truly christened me the* Green Goddess. *I certainly didn't agree!*

It was a family joke that I was a 'Friday Nighter', made up of odd parts, and they'd forgotten to add my boobs. My mother – a pretty, nicely proportioned four foot eleven – had called me a freak when, in my early teens, I shot up to become a lanky five foot ten. My father used to call me Whippet. I decided, secretly, that when I was grown up I would make enough money to pay for an operation to remove two inches from my long upper thighs, which would make me a normal height. What a gruesome thought!

At about thirteen I developed a stoop and hunched my shoulders, so no one could see my 'deformity'. How I envied all my friends with their lovely figures. I only wanted to hide mine. I was all out of proportion, and it made me very shy and insecure.

I was taller than my brother, who was three years older than me, and taller than most of the boys in my year at school. But I was bright, and could be clever if my attention was caught. I was also very athletic. The long legs, at least, won me many a race, and gradually over the years I developed my confidence and physique through sport.

By fifteen I was girl captain of the house sports team and the school athletic team, and was winning races everywhere. I played a mean game of tennis and was vice-captain of the school tennis team too. I was good at the high jump and the hurdles, and was always the speedy last post in the successful relay team. I had the opportunity and ability to excel.

On one occasion, representing the county, I lined up, confident as ever, at the start of the hundred yards. In my borrowed spikes – my father wouldn't give me the money for my own – I shot off as the gun fired. But this time it was different. A powerful young woman raced past me to win with ease. Her name was Mary Bignal, from Millfield School in Somerset, and some years later, in 1964, she was to become the Olympic champion under her married name of Mary Rand.

At times like that, over-confidence gets sorted out and one gets well and truly put in one's place. But in fact I never forgot those awful, awkward years before I discovered how to turn my physique to advantage, and I think this is where some of my sympathetic nature comes from. Throughout my life, whatever my work has been, I've tried to help and encourage those less fortunate or shy or handicapped, mentally or physically.

I left school (truly the happiest days of my life) at sixteen with seven O levels and a scholarship to the West of England College of Art. I desperately wanted to learn fashion and design, or to train as an art teacher. I was torn between that and teaching gym. But my father said I was to train for a 'proper' job. He *sent me to the College of Commerce in Bristol, and I hated it.*

Saturday, 11 June

My birthday. I'm forty-nine today, and I have to admit the events of the past month do make me feel one year older.

We came down to Mudeford late last night and now, at breakfast time, Nic has arrived. He's come from Bristol for the weekend and has a delightful girlfriend with him, Charlotte. I realize I know her parents from my days in Bristol and laugh as she reminds me that her father, an orthodontist, removed all my wisdom teeth many years ago. Peter has gone to fetch Holly, his fourteen-year-old daughter, from Winchester. He was divorced many years ago but sees Holly regularly.

I open my cards and presents. I'm already wearing mine from Peter, my pretty pink and turquoise tracksuit from Florida. Nic has brought a beautiful, slightly oriental, square-shaped china vase, decorated with magnolia and exotic birds. It's a present from both boys, and I'm delighted with it. Peter returns with Holly, who with a twinkle in her eye gives me a box of dark chocolate brazils, which she knows I can't resist.

Peter and his willing helpers decide to launch the boat. It's a small Dory, and they're soon speeding off across the harbour. I think back to when the boys were small. . . .

At school Nic was the more competent sportsman, although both were good all-rounders. He played an excellent game of squash and was part of the successful Avon county team. Like his brother, he was to become a keen sailor, and I recall delivering him to the Island Cruising Club in Salcombe in Devon one Easter for the holiday sailing course. The winter had been severe and Easter was early that year. Putting him, aged eight, complete with his kitbag aboard the small craft that was to take him to his floating base for the next week, I had a pang of conscience. There was plenty of snow and ice still

around, and I knew he would have to do capsize drill. But he
returned home one week later having loved every minute, and
it increased his already strong interest and ability in sailing.

The weather is beautiful, so we decide today is the day to buy a
barbecue. Hopefully, if the weather stays like today, we can use
it many times. At the local garden centre we all have differing
opinions as to what will be the ideal model for our small walled
garden. Decision finally made, we rush home and get it going.
Nic is the chef and lunch is excellent, if a little charred.

Afterwards, Nic and Charlotte take themselves off on our
Raleigh Maverick all-terrain bikes. Peter and I cycle a lot and
find them ideal for this part of the country, because we can use
them on forest paths and beaches as well as roads. Holly and
her father clean down the boat and put it away safely in the
garage, and late in the afternoon he takes her to Christchurch
Station to catch the train home. It's the first time Holly's done
this alone. How she's grown up in the few years I've known her.

While he's gone, there's a ring on the door bell. Marion and
Pete Squires, local friends, have sent me a beautiful flower
arrangement for my birthday. I'm thrilled.

They join us, early in the evening, along with our friend
David Burton and his smart wife Rhonda. Peter cracks a bottle
of bubbly and everyone toasts me. We move off to a local
French restaurant where we eat merrily and converse noisily.
It's a happy evening and we round it off with a Green God-
dess crème de menthe cocktail. As everyone drinks my health
I silently resolve to make fifty.

Sunday, 12 June

One of the joys of Mudeford is the sandbank, which can be
reached from the quayside by a small ferry boat. Arriving at
the jetty, you land on a thin finger of sand lined on either side
with some five hundred wooden huts, a remnant of Victorian
times. The huts are a discreet place to change in for swimming

or sailing, and their owners can take cover in them when the weather gets bad. But they also provide carefree and very cosy holiday homes for many families, complete with bunk beds and cooking facilities. Life is simple and unsophisticated on the sandbank and you have to make your own entertainment. Most of the huts have no running water and the loos are communal. There are no cars because it is simply a bank of sand. Huts on the one side look into Mudeford harbour and on up to the town of Christchurch. On the other side they look out over Highcliffe bay and towards the Isle of Wight.

David and Rhonda own one of the huts and from time to time give a barbecue on the sandbank. Friends often take food and drink to help out, and if the weather is fine arrive in their own canoes or small boats, or on surfboards. But today we all take the safer way, the ferry.

I help Rhonda prepare the food while David takes Peter and the other guests for a spin in his new Bayliner boat. Peter is envious, and when he comes back talks of buying one himself. They were half the price in America.

Back at the house, I'm amused to see two amateur artists have set up their easels on the grass in front of our house and are painting the beautiful view I had described on *Something to Treasure*. I ring the artist, Christopher Hollick, who thanks me for the exposure and tells me that some of his work has been selected for exhibition at the Royal Academy this year. The amateur artists continue for several hours. I smile to myself and am secretly pleased there were some viewers out there.

Meanwhile, Peter has slipped off to walk down into the village and visit his mother. Poor man – he needs someone to talk to, someone who can give him support. I remember Mr Scott's words on the subject only a few days ago. Nic and Charlotte leave early in the evening to drive back to Bristol, and I take the opportunity of an early night.

Monday, 13 June

A lot has happened in one month, and I've learnt so much about cancer and its treatment.

Peter returns to London by the early train. At ten o'clock he rings to say he's very sick. He's been to the office but he's now back in the flat. Could it be a reaction?

Before he left this morning, he confessed he had told Pete, over the weekend, that I had a problem and Pete in turn told his wife, Marion. This morning she invites me for a girls' talk at her bungalow in the village. She tells me that Pete, a builder in his late forties, is not well himself. He has a heart problem and an ulcer. She's very sympathetic and understands when I tell her I may have cancer. Together we share our worries.

Leaving her, I decide to be more practical and prepare for the future. I would like to convalesce in Mudeford, in which case I will need some help. Peter doesn't have a washing machine, so I must buy one. I arrange to have it delivered during the week; Peter's mother will see it in if I can't be there. As I drive back to London I wonder if Ken, a retired local man who has done odd jobs for us in the past, would be able to help if I need physical assistance around the house. I must ask him. But who can I ask to help me in the flat in London immediately I come out of hospital? Virginia, a Filipino, comes in to clean for me, but I can hardly ask her to fetch and carry for a semi-invalid, and in any case she's only here one day a week. I'll have to think of something else.

Tuesday, 14 June

Peter says he's better this morning, but I've woken up feeling very angry and resentful. This damn cancer. I desperately need some support today – I do wish Tim would ring me. Perhaps he isn't very concerned. I don't want to make a fuss and have the family flapping unnecessarily, but a phone call or a letter would be a comfort and make me feel a bit more loved.

As I look through my morning post I find John, my ex, has sent a lovely birthday card. We always remember each other's birthdays, and exchange cards and gifts at Christmas. We also write one another postcards when we go away on holiday. I think I'll phone him. He's sympathetic as ever, but tells me Tim is very busy at work. John has seen him recently and assures me that Tim *is* concerned. Even so, why can't he at least give me a quick phone call? But enough of these thoughts – I've a lunch party today with Patsy Wilcox, my ex-producer from *Breakfast Time*.

It's a splendid gathering, mostly presenters, producers and back-scene bods from *The Money Programme*, which Patsy has recently been working on. As I talk to her producer the stimulating conversation gives me an idea, and a concept for a new programme emerges which could involve my interest in art. I resolve to put the idea down on paper when I get home. The trouble is I'm always doing this. Over the years I've sent lots of ideas off to TV producers, who in turn have pinched the ideas or part of them. Then a year or so later I've seen them as the basis of a so-called new programme. It's maddening, but it happens to me and my colleagues all the time and is one of the hazards of our business. I decide to keep this particular idea to myself; then, when I'm over my imminent troubles and strong enough, I'll try to progress it. For the meantime it can go in my 'good ideas' file along with the others.

The other guests say goodbye and return to work, which leaves Patsy, a close friend of hers and myself alone. We busy ourselves clearing up. Patsy asks me how the boys are, and can sense I'm a bit uptight. She is someone I know I can trust, so I decide to confide in her, and it makes me feel more at ease. As we wash up, we talk about the problems all women face as they get older. We despair at the increasing number of our friends, workmates and families who have been through distress of this sort. It upsets us all, and we feel strongly that more must be done to research into and prevent this wretched disease.

Back home, prospects of work slip by. Working freelance, it haunts me to turn away good jobs. But Annie and I have to refuse work, saying I'll be away and unfortunately not available for a few weeks. Anxiously, I hope my money will see me through this crisis. Over the years I've put some aside for a rainy day, but I didn't bargain on this storm.

When I was talking to John this morning, he reminded me it was twenty years ago in July that I had my first operation for the removal of some lumps in my throat. And that was when I started to get involved in keep-fit.

Marriage and babies, combined with a lack of babysitters, ended the regular exercising and training I had enjoyed as a teenager, but I naturally kept trim by walking the children and doing plenty of gardening. Even hanging out the washing, stretching up and down, was excellent exercise. Running up and down the stairs, coping with toddlers, was good for the whole body.

However, as our children begin to grow up we adults get crafty and lazy, and use our brains instead of our brawn with labour-saving devices. By twenty-nine my lifestyle was not so healthy, and when I found myself in hospital and confined to bed after surgery – first a partial thyroidectomy to deal with the lumps in my throat, and then an emergency operation for appendicitis – I had time to think about myself.

I realized I had gradually neglected my health. I was doing less exercise, and had fallen into bad eating habits as so many young mums do. I was eating too much. I'd become the family dustbin, polishing off the left-overs and sampling the cakes, and I was hooked on sweets and chocolate. As a result, I had become lethargic. My body was out of tune, I was overweight, and my skin wasn't all that bright.

Curiously, it didn't affect my work as a model particularly. It meant I modelled size fourteen rather than size twelve, but that was almost an asset – outside London, there were far more comfortable size fourteens than there were anorexic size tens, and the customers wanted to see the clothes on someone their own size. In any case, when you're five foot ten, like me, you can get away with a lot – and pancake make-up does wonders with a chocolate-bar complexion!

But it didn't feel right, so I decided to do something to help myself, not only for my own good but also for the sake of the family.

After a lot of research into diet and exercise, and with a great deal of determination, I realized and felt the benefits of a healthy, balanced diet with lots of fibre. Combined with a simple exercise programme, it became my lifestyle.

Feeling fit, as I usually do, makes me glad to be alive and full of energy. I'm more able to cope with the stresses and strains of my everyday life. Nowadays tennis, sailing, swimming, cycling and a weekly work-out are my ways of keeping fit. Skiing's my favourite form of exercise, but being so expensive, unfortunately, it's not often possible.

Apparently my new-found enthusiasm proved infectious as far as my girlfriends and my model girl workmates were concerned. Before very long I was giving impromptu lessons backstage, which eventually became official keep-fit classes.

Butlin's saw the start of my teaching keep-fit in public about eighteen years ago. I was part of a national promotional campaign for the Outline Slimming Bureau, to be called An Outline to Living. It was my fashion expertise and organizing abilities for which I had been brought in. The team also included experts on diet, nutrition and cooking, and all of us attended a keep-fit course over several weeks in London. I loved it, having just a few years previously rediscovered the joys of exercising.

A week before we set off to Butlin's in Minehead for the start of the summer campaign, I asked the boss what form the keep-fit class would take and who would lead it. She replied she had been waiting for a natural to emerge from the team – and it was me.

I made my preparations the night before the big day and nervously met Brett Cresswell, Butlin's Entertainment Manager, at Minehead. He taught me how to use the technical equipment, and invited me to watch him on stage that evening to pick up tips on how to handle an audience. I learnt quickly. Next morning we all dressed in red leotards and tights, got out and got on. It was an instant success, and one I was to repeat every year for Butlin's, and later Pontin's, at holiday camps in Wales and the West Country.

I owe my success to healthy living. I decided all those years ago that I had to look after my body, because it was the place in which I lived. I exercised and maintained my mobility as the years advanced, and improved my circulation, heart and lung functions. And I find that feeling better makes me look better.

Now that the pain has been largely removed from keep-fit classes around the country, we can all thankfully get back to the feeling of exhilaration and not exhaustion from exercise classes. Working on Breakfast Time, as the Green Goddess, gave me the unique opportunity to meet people of all types and all ages from many walks of life all around Britain. It delighted me to see the pleasure derived by so many ordinary people who exercised regularly in some form or another – either quite simply at home, or in controlled groups at keep-fit classes and in sports centres. Many of those same enthusiastic people told me of their joy in discovering a better, healthier life. They'd changed their diets, they exercised more, they'd cut out smoking, they'd controlled their drink and drug problems. They felt as if they'd been given a second chance in life and were enjoying it.

For my part, through exercise I want to encourage people to take advantage of living their lives to the full. To encourage them to use their bodies as nature intended – to keep them strong and supple. The body is a beautiful machine given to us free, yet so many people abuse it. I always remember one elderly lady, who had exercised for many years with the Keep Fit Association, saying to me, 'Diana, if you don't use it, you may lose it.' She was talking about her own healthy body. She was seventy-five and she had certainly kept her health, mobility and therefore her independence into old age.

Wednesday, 15 June

Preparing the monthly expenses is my most unfavourite job but it has to be done, says my accountant, Philip, in Birmingham who tries to keep me in order. Being self-employed means I must keep a strict record of everything I earn and every penny I spend, from travel expenses to paper clips, in the pursuit of my career. I suppose I'm a bit of a jack of all trades, with my work in television, presentation, fashion and journalism. I lead a complicated life which is always varied but never dull, and I wouldn't have it any differently.

A surprise telephone call from Tim breaks the monotony of the figure work. I'm delighted he's phoned. He sounds well, but very busy with his work. I listen as he tells me his news. He doesn't ask me how I am, but I sound bright and I know he's probably thinking that no particular news from me must be good news. I tell him I'd like to visit him next week, and he suggests Wednesday evening. Privately I think it's a case of taking the mountain to Mohammed, but it makes me feel happier.

Thursday, 16 June

Lunch with one of my favourite men today – a belated birthday treat. Christopher Price has arranged to meet me at Ciboure, a pleasant French restaurant in Eccleston Street, Belgravia.

We've been close friends for twenty years, having first met when we were both modelling clothes part-time for two very upmarket shops in Stratford-upon-Avon, in Warwickshire. I was a young mum from Bristol with small children, and I fitted my work around school time and family commitments. Chris, with his blond hair and blue eyes, was constantly being poached from his job in Birmingham for the occasional appearance on the catwalk or in front of the camera.

We're both very tall and we made a good couple. His boyish sense of fun complemented my keen sense of humour, and over the years we've developed a deep and trusting relationship – nothing sexual, but very caring. I regard him as one of my closest and dearest friends – he's always such a tonic to be with.

Fifteen years ago, he moved to London, where nowadays he runs a successful public relations company. At the start of my rise to stardom as the Green Goddess, Chris came to my rescue. I did not have an agent, and overnight he stepped into the gap, putting himself between me and the press and business offers which were suddenly flooding in. Having already signed a contract with the BBC which made me exclusive to them, I was unable to accept most of the offers. But he dealt with them and arranged interviews with the hungry press. He and his assistant, Rosemary, negotiated contracts for the first book, record, cassettes and videos. He also dealt with all my other business commitments, until finally it became too much for him and I found myself a professional agent.

His mother, Liz, was a darling. A wizard with figures, she became my book-keeper and helped me with my wretched accounts, which she knew I loathed. Sadly, she died of cancer two years ago.

Because of his mother, I can see Christopher is terribly upset as I tell him my news. However, it's my birthday treat so we try to put our cares aside. Chris says he knows I'm good at public relations, and to my delight and surprise invites me to consider joining him in his expanding business after my operation, should I decide to change or not be able to pursue my present career. What a wonderful offer. I know we could work well together and in conjunction with Rosemary, now his partner and another of my closest pals. We toast our futures.

As we finish lunch, Chris asks me whether I realize that another friend of ours, Elizabeth, had a mastectomy some years ago. I certainly do not, but I'm very interested to hear about it and ask Chris if he can arrange for me to talk to her. I badly want to speak to someone who has experienced the operation, and want to know how she is. Christopher tells me she's wonderfully well.

Back in the flat, I'm excited to hear my brother's voice on the phone after so many years. He's received my letter telling him of the proposed operation, and now I tell him about the possibility of reconstruction. 'Oh!' he laughs. 'So you're having a silicone job, are you?' That makes me feel tetchy, but I suppose I'm being over-sensitive – and at heart I'm happy he's phoned and is interested in my welfare. I wonder if he'll visit me soon – that would be nice. His manner is a little brusque, like my father's was, and the conversation is somewhat awkward and stilted. I feel very emotional, and think back to when we were young and such good chums. What a pity my divorce has pushed us apart. Perhaps things will be better from now on.

My mind begins to wander a little, and I recall our early childhood in a small Somerset village between Bristol and Weston-super-Mare . . .

Our parents both came from the Bristol area, but decided to move out and rear their family in the country. I was a war baby, born in 1939, but we saw nothing of it in the country. My early schooldays were spent at the small, traditional Church of England school in the village of Backwell. It stood on a hill at the top of Dark Lane, near the lovely Norman church where we children had been christened and which we attended every Sunday. My brother, being three years older than myself, was already at school when I started, and on my big day I walked eagerly hand in hand with him up Dark Lane, where he delivered me to Mr Branch, the headmaster. I very soon made friends, including one of Mr Branch's own children, who were fondly referred to as his twiglets.

The playground led into a vegetable garden, probably Mr Branch's, and a path through it led up to the woods on Backwell Hill. In this garden and the woods beyond I saw birds, rabbits, moles and pink, spineless baby hedgehogs. I learnt to recognize the flowers of the hedgerow, the trees and the shrubs. I would

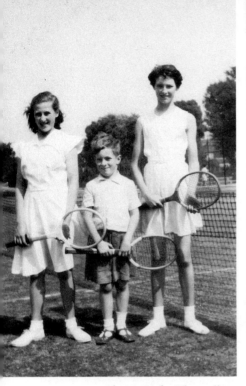

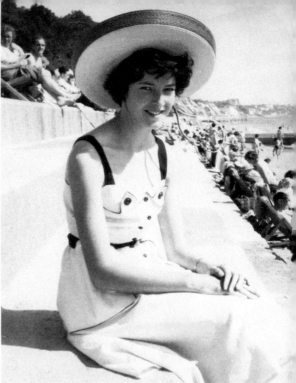

Above Left: The tallest one on the tennis court.
Above right: Growing up self-consciously.
Below: Training to be a personnel officer.

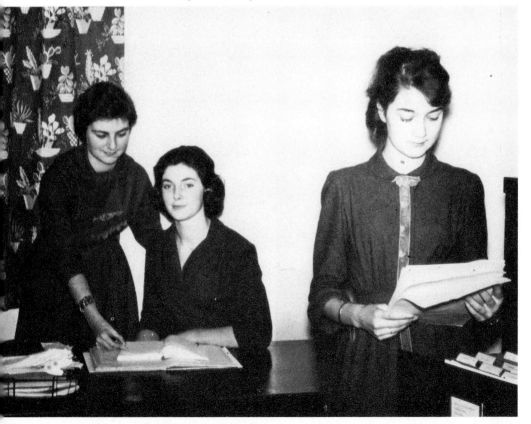

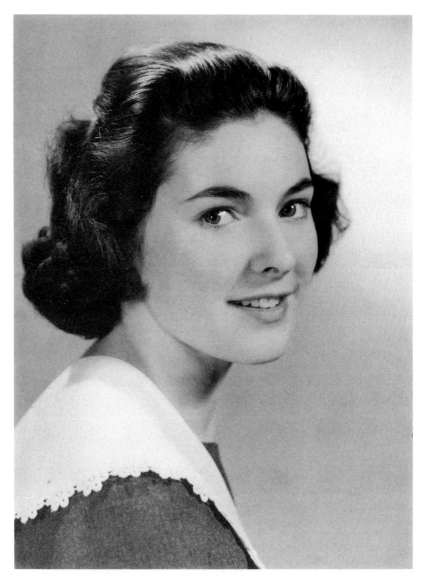

Me aged eighteen. (Courtesy Bromhead of Bristol.)

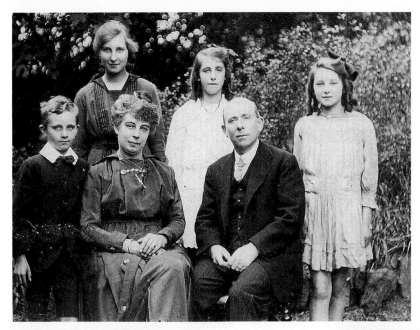

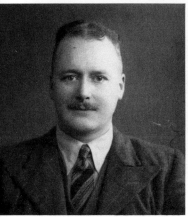

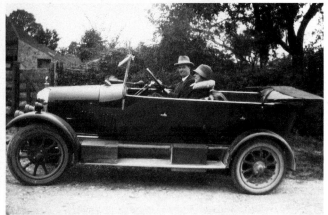

Top: My mother's family: (seated) Granny and Grandpa Snell; (standing from left to right) Uncle Ken, Aunt Phyllis, Aunt Kathleen, my mother.
Above left: My father.
Above right: My father's parents: Granny and Grandpa Dicker.
Right: My mother.

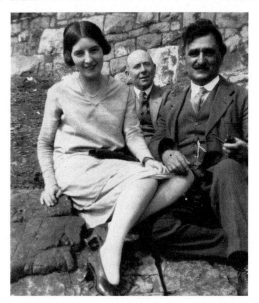

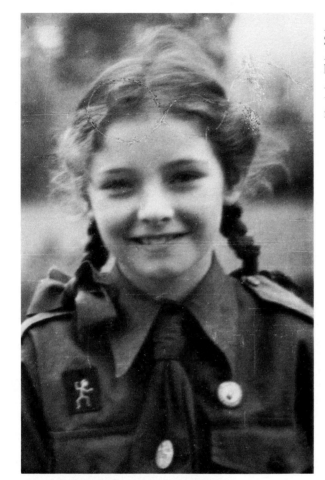

Left: Me as a Brownie Sprite.
Below Left: With my brother Anthony.
Below right: On holiday with Anthony and my father in Boscombe.

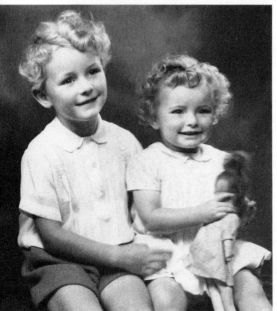

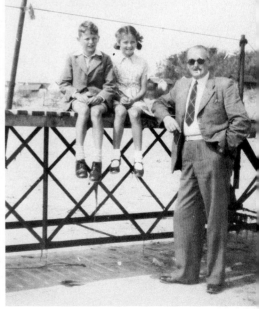

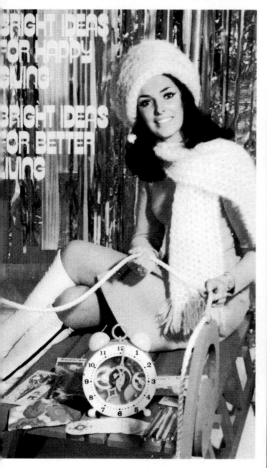

Above: Adding a touch of glamour.
(Courtesy Bright Ideas Ltd.)
Right: Helping the family firm. (Courtesy
Desmond Tripp.)

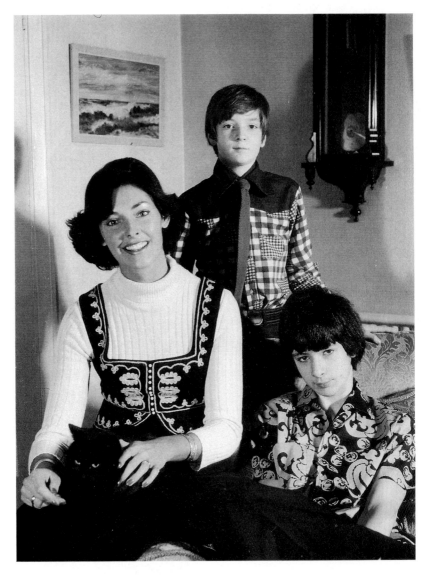

With Poppy the cat and the boys.

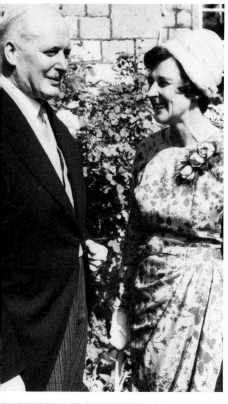

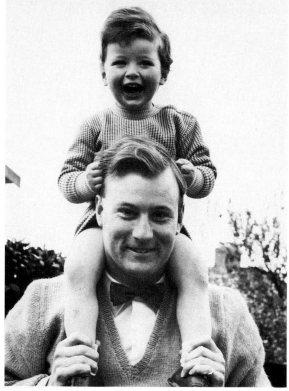

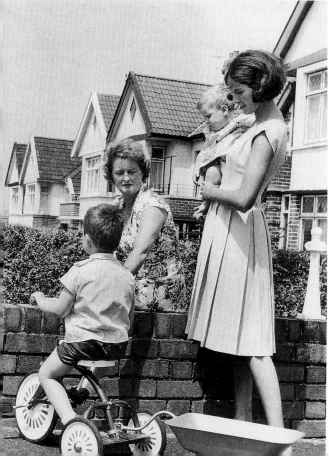

Above left: Father and his sister, my Aunt Mona, at my wedding.
Above right: Tim with my husband John.
Left: Me with Tim and baby Nic. (Courtesy Bristol Evening Post.)

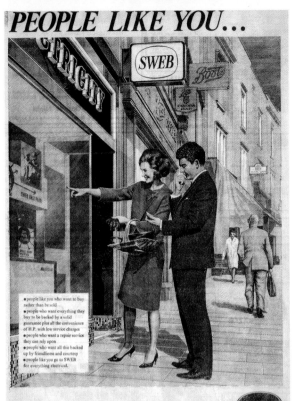

My first photographic modelling assignment.
(Courtesy Bristol Evening Post.)

Down to basics in the sixties.
(Courtesy Morses.)

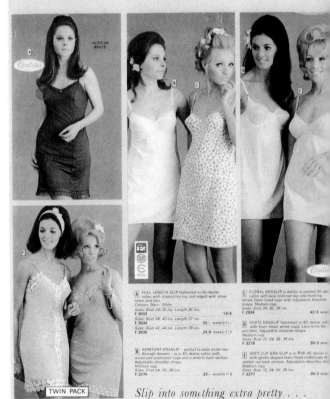

wander off, later to be found painstakingly searching for wild strawberries to take home to my mother. I discovered the dark paths beyond the yew hedges, massed with violets in spring. And I remember the excitement of walking to school in winter through the deep snowdrifts, and the unpleasantness of returning home cold, wet and miserable in the pouring rain.

One spring, I was chosen by the school to be May Queen. A traditional maypole was erected in the playground, and our teacher, Mrs Nicholls, spent hours teaching us the intricacies of the traditional May dance. Attached to the top of the maypole were lots of long, coloured ribbons. Each child took hold of one and, on command and in time to the music, one group of children skipped in one direction in and out of the others coming the other way. The idea was to avoid a collision. In the process the ribbons became woven tightly together and formed a pretty pattern down the pole. The theory was good, but it took hours of practice and lots of Mrs Nicholls' patience to get it right.

However, on May Day all was well, and I did my bit proudly wearing my crown which Mrs Nicholls and my mother had made from a gold cake frill and dozens of tiny pink miniature rosebuds. It was my first public performance and I enjoyed it – I must have been good because I was asked back again the next year!

But our home life was more formal and less jolly, strongly influenced by my father. A tall, upright, good-looking, well-disciplined man, he commuted daily by car to his job as sales manager for an oil refinery in Bristol. To his annoyance and disbelief, he had been found medically unfit for active service in 1939 with a heart complaint, so he spent the war years doing his bit as a special constable in the village.

My brother and I were frightened of him. He was very dictatorial, extremely strict almost to the point of cruelty, and not easy to communicate with. Over the years he became even more difficult. My childhood memories of him are of my nervousness and desire not to upset him. He insisted that we were brought up like Victorian children, to be seen and not heard. If we were naughty, we were always punished, and I remember all too often being sent up to my room for hours on end with the backs of my legs smarting from the cane that he had put across them as I ran up the stairs. I don't think I was ever really naughty at all—just high-spirited. We soon learnt to duck and dive him, however, and because he was a man of such disciplined regularity it was possible to enjoy ourselves most of the time, but to come firmly back in line when he was about.

My mother, whom we adored, played the same game. She was one of us, and we learnt to clock-watch from an early age and to know when to rein in. A pretty little woman, artistic, quick and capable, she too was high-spirited. Sometimes this would bubble over when we were sitting very formally— as we did, each evening and weekend—around the dining table. All too often, the nervous tension would be relieved by a word or a look across the well-mannered table. It doesn't take much to make me, a compulsive giggler, start off, particularly when the air is thick with repression. When this happened, my mother, with her infectious sense of humour, would start to giggle as well.

These occasions would usually end in tears, with one or all of us being sent out of the room by a furious father who did not see the joke. I think he was as hard on my mother as he was on us, but he was her life and she did everything he wanted. She had never been out to work, and never learnt to express her own personality. She was dominated by him. But she was a wonderful mother and a close friend to us children.

Tragically, as a girl of sixteen, I was to find her one lunchtime collapsed and unconscious in the bathroom. She had been decorating for days, papering the hallway, and that morning she was painting the banisters. The paint was still wet, the can and brush on the floor. I thought she had choked, and tried to clear her throat—but she only groaned. In terror and panic I rushed to fetch a neighbour, and soon an ambulance was on its way.

They took her away. But the red fluff from the blankets caught on the wet paint and was to stay there for months as a painful reminder of the worst day of my life. I telephoned my father at work. He didn't return till we children had gone to bed. He had been to the hospital. He came quietly into our rooms and awkwardly told us she would not be coming back. She was dead. She had had a cerebral haemorrhage and never recovered. She was forty-seven. Life was never the same again. I'd lost my best friend and my childhood was over. Oh, my God, how I've missed her over the years. And I miss her now.

Friday, 17 June

I take a taxi to the offices of *Shropshire Life*, the publishers of *Pinnacle*, the Rolls Royce enthusiasts' magazine. With the art editor, I select the appropriate photographs from my New Forest photographic session to complement my editorial. I hope *Look Good, Feel Great* is shaping up as well – I should have the proofs soon.

Work is rolling in, but I'm having to fend it off. Earlier in the year I agreed to help organize a national series of one hundred work-outs in aid of Help the Aged. They're pressing for dates and I've had to delay my first public appearance, which they would have liked in September or October. We agree a date in November, and I set that as my goal for getting going again with a public keep-fit session, scheduled to go on for a maximum of a hundred minutes. I must be back on form by then. I postpone a video, planned for July or August, in which I was to have done some physical movements, and I begin to worry again about my finances. How long will I be out of action? I take an overall look at my financial position and begin to work out a contingency plan.

I telephone the claims department of my private health scheme and ask them what I can expect in the way of reimbursement of the hospital charges and surgeons' fees. I hope the major part of the bill will be the scheme's responsibility. I'm not convinced, however, and there seems to be some doubt because the hospital is in London and the charges are higher than the scale I'm paying for.

I know my cancer would have been treated promptly on the National Health, but as a freelance I feel it's worth paying for private health care so that I'm not kept out of work if something more routine goes wrong, and I have to wait for treatment. At the moment, too, privacy is essential – if the press find out what's wrong I'm terrified no one will want to offer me work even when I'm better. I have to preserve my image of perfect health.

Supper is in good company this evening at the Bombay Brasserie off the Gloucester Road with Audrey and Chris Dunning, whom we last saw at the opening of their daughter Stephanie's shop. They are exuberant, having taken possession of their new boat, *Marionette*, this morning in Ipswich. Chris, an experienced yachtsman, was captain of the successful British Admiral's Cup team in 1977, and more recently captain of the British team which won the Sardinia Cup for the first time in 1986. He is an inspiration to be with, having with great determination overcome severe physical disabilities as a result of polio when he was a boy. I listen with admiration to his tales of adventures in conditions which would deter all but the strongest of sailors.

Then Peter and Chris discuss business, whilst Audrey and I talk about more personal things. She understands.

Saturday, 18 June

The weather this morning is beautiful, sunny and warm. Good conditions for the annual show on Putney Common, where I'm doing a sponsored public keep-fit session in the main arena to raise funds for Help the Aged – a kind of rehearsal for the series I'm doing for them later in the year. But there isn't a very good turn-out for my session – I don't think the publicity has been organized very effectively. Never mind: the performance must be the same despite the small numbers.

I've given the charity a large quantity of my book *Get Fit with the Green Goddess*, which they can sell to help swell their funds. I spend my time between sessions chatting up the public, selling my books and signing my autographs for 10p a time. Every little helps. Several military personnel come up and say hello. They will be appearing in the main arena later. They look so smart, and remind me that we all worked together last July at the Royal Tournament at Earls Court.

What an experience that was. Each year one of the services is featured prominently, and in 1987 it was the turn of the Royal Navy. I had been 'adopted' by the Navy as part of their display team, and as a consequence became the Blue Goddess for a month.

At the end of the first half the team was featured in historical costume, and performed the sailors' hornpipe to the delight of the huge crowds. Getting faster and faster, the dance built up to a crescendo of sound and movement, with the audience clapping in time to or, more often, in advance of the music. As the lads stood to receive their applause, the Blue Goddess was announced. I burst into the arena, ran into the middle and was promptly hoisted aloft a large capstan.

I invited the audience to come on down to join the sailors and me as we danced the hornpipe. They didn't need much encouragement – they came in their thousands, thundering down the steps and jumping over the terraces. Boys, girls, mums, dads and even grandads, often old sailors just wanting to show off their dancing skills to their families. After a quick lesson from me, they reeled and rocked in time to the music. The young lads of the team encouraged everyone, but most particularly the pretty girls, to join in the fun.

After a few minutes' chaos I changed the tempo, and, with the music jazzed up by the splendid Royal Marine band, I had the whole audience clapping in time as we jumped into action with a modern work-out.

For me, high up on my perch, it was a splendid sight. I could see the entire arena bending, swaying, jumping and clapping at my command. I had a feeling of power, and I felt very proud of our performance. I was even more proud to find myself in the line-up being presented at the end of each show to the visiting

VIP, who took the salute. It was often a member of the Royal Family. My favourite Royal at the Tournament was the Queen Mother, who seemed to have thoroughly enjoyed every minute of the show.

Sunday, 19 June

Another beautiful day, and we're back in Mudeford again. It was worth making the effort to come down last night just to be able to stand in the window this morning and watch the activity in the harbour. It's busy with small craft, bobbing and glinting in the sunshine, and surfers with their lovely, colourful sails. Nowhere beats England on a day like today.

Marion and Pete phone us and we decide to take advantage of the weather and go over to Yarmouth for the day on the Isle of Wight ferry. Members of our local sailing club in Christchurch are visiting the club there to take part in a day of competition races. It seems like a good excuse for a day out in the sun.

We join Marion and Pete and then meet up with Rhonda and David to drive to Lymington, where we board the Sealink ferry. As we lean on the top deck rail we look out enviously over the thousands of magnificent craft moored in the marina. Many of them are alive with people busily hoisting sails or starting up engines, preparing for a day at sea. Large boats like these are a rarity in Mudeford and Christchurch, because the waters are too shallow for them to make a safe passage into the harbour.

Marion and Pete think of their own sailing boat, which left Lymington marina earlier this year to be sailed down to the Mediterranean. They will join it there in a few weeks' time for a holiday in the sun. Lucky them.

The water is calm and the thirty-minute crossing smooth. Peter has decided to bring a smile to everyone's face – from my large hold-all he produces the plastic champagne flutes we had in Florida, and ceremoniously arranges them on top of a life-raft. Then, with aplomb, he opens a surprise bottle of champagne which he has brought with him. The six of us, outrageously and much to the amusement of our fellow passengers, drink it with style, as if we started every day this way!

Peter and I feel very close, and our happiness is shared by our friends. We walk and talk, wander through the pretty, quaint streets of Yarmouth, and then have lunch at the club house. In the afternoon we sit in the sunshine on the patio and watch the racing.

One of the races is for the single-handed sailing boats called scows; Peter and David get enthusiastic, and decide they will buy a scow to share between them. For the next few hours they enquire about second-hand boats. The rest of us wonder how, if they are successful, we will ever get it back to Christchurch. We know they aren't capable of sailing it back; nevertheless Hunt the Boat becomes the exercise of the day. But we don't have to deal with that particular problem; their quest is unsuccessful, and we return to Christchurch without a boat. However, they then head immediately for the sailing club to scan the notice boards there. Again, without success. Secretly I wonder if Peter will have much opportunity to sail this season – let alone me. Ah well, there's always next year.

Back at home I feel tired and try to sleep, but suddenly I'm frightened. I'm still unnerved at the prospect of my imminent operation and how it may change our lives. Peter senses my concern, puts his arms around me and consoles me.

Monday, 20 June

Peter is up and off back to London at 5.30 a.m. I'm calmer today, and feel peaceful as I garden and clean up the house. The new washing machine is delivered and plumbed in – it will be a great help when I come down to convalesce. I box up Maggie, who has exhausted herself trying to catch butterflies in the garden all day, and drive back to London.

Peter has been to see his doctor about his heart, which has been causing him concern for the past few weeks. A faulty valve is the cause. He's told he must avoid stress, but pills can keep the problem in check. I must be putting him under extra strain, and it makes me feel guilty. Over the past few years he has been the one who has needed a little support from me, the strong one, and now the tables have been turned. I know my problem is probably more serious than Peter's, so in many ways I'm the one who really needs the support – but it's my nature to give support, rather than receive it, and I find it hard to change that even now.

Peter has explained my situation to his doctor, who, in return, assures him that my specialist has an excellent reputation and that I will be well cared for.

Tuesday, 21 June

The surgeons have said they may operate at the end of the month. I decide to forget work, and ring the agency to tell them so. Bother the money. I want time to see my friends and family. I'll put my flat in order and do all the odd jobs I've been meaning to do for months. I'll plant flowers in the tubs and troughs on my balcony, so that when I come home from hospital they'll be pretty and colourful. I'll enjoy doing that, and it'll help me relax. And I'll do the same in Mudeford next weekend.

I start to plan my travels. I've so much to fit in, and so many people to see. Can I bear the emotion of going back to my beautiful home in Bristol, where I spent my married years, and seeing John again?

Wednesday, 22 June

I'm up early and off to the dentist. He wishes me luck with the operation – he must know how I feel. Then I walk to Sloane Square, and in Peter Jones buy some odds and ends I may need. Back home I pack my hospital case. That done, I prepare for my trip to the country and look up my routes to Dartmouth in Devon, my first port of call.

Just as I'm about to walk out of the door the phone rings. It's Elizabeth, and her voice is music to my ears. She says she understands the trauma I'm going through and suggests we meet early next week, on my return. She will be mentally alongside me through it all, she says. It sounds as if my fairy godmother has appeared, and I feel choked with repressed emotion as she tells me that my planned journey to the West Country will be difficult. She warns me of the black thoughts and sad moments I'll have visiting those close to me, but asks me to be strong and cheerful for their sake. Elizabeth's call reassures me, and I set off in good spirits to tackle Tim.

The weather is superb. Devon and Somerset have never looked so wonderful, and I'm filled with nostalgia.

I arrive at Tim's flat in the centre of Dartmouth, behind the market square. A tall, strong young man, he's looking well. Friends say he looks like me, but you can never see such likenesses yourself. His hair is dark, as mine was before I went blonde, and he looks tanned from all the sailing he does. His naval lieutenant's uniform suits him and he wears the gold dolphins – indicating he's a submariner – with pride. And I feel equally proud to be his mum. He's worked hard all his life, at school, Dartmouth and university, to get where he is.

I sense he feels awkward with me this afternoon, so I set about the task of clearing up his flat and tackling the mountain of ironing stacked in the corner. Nothing changes! I find the situation easier once I'm doing something – I'm more relaxed, and he responds.

Jill, his girlfriend, is being examined on her PhD tomorrow and he's anxious for her. She phones from Birmingham University and I hear them talk. She's nervous, but I'm secretly confident she'll be OK. She's a smart girl.

I enquire if marriage is in the pipeline. He tells me they have no plans and prefer it that way. They both have ambitions, careers and changes planned for the next few years.

Chores finished, Tim drives us to a country pub where, over

a glass of wine, we both feel more comfortable with each other. He asks me how I am, but can already see from my optimism and cheerfulness that I'm all right. Back in Dartmouth we go to a small local restaurant run by a friend, who makes us both welcome. It's good to be together and I feel happy I've made the long journey down to Devon and can share a little of his life.

Gradually, as I ask him about his work and his career plans, he opens up. He's not self-centred, but I know he won't be able to broach the subject of my cancer himself, so I lead into it myself, in a sensible, matter-of-fact way. His concern shows as he prompts me to fill in details. I sense that Tim, like so many people, may feel that cancer is final, that it's synonymous with death. And that's why I want to tell him the truth, to fill his head with facts, not myths.

Sleep comes more easily tonight. I'm quite content.

Thursday, 23 June

I'm wakened by the town clock striking and the crashing of milk crates in the dairy opposite. Tim is up early, and after breakfast together he's off up the hill to the college to organize his students. He returns after an hour or so and together we walk in the hot sunshine, doing a whirlwind tour of the town. I buy equipment for my new barbecue in a local shop, but all too soon it's time to kiss each other goodbye.

Quickly I get into my car and drive off before Tim can see my tears. I have sensed his deep emotion, and realize that behind the tough façade is the same sensitive child I used to know. Naval training and life in general have taught him to cover up his feelings, and living at sea aboard his submarine for days on end has naturally hardened him.

As I drive through the countryside I think back over those precious years of childhood that flew by so quickly. . . .

John and I had prepared the boys to be independent, but how difficult I'd found it to let go the apron strings. I had been against the idea of them going to boarding school at seven, as John had done, and said so again at nine and eleven. As a child I had experienced the loss of my mother, and I was well aware of the effect it had had on my own life. I wanted the boys to be there with me, at home, throughout their schooldays and until they were old enough to be set free into the world. I wanted them to have both parents to rely on, to talk to, to tell their troubles to daily. In return we could encourage them, know their needs, their friends and, more importantly, what they were getting up to.

Through the years it had worked well, and both Tim and Nic had grown up to be good, strong, intelligent individuals whom John and I were justly pleased with and liked as people. But how painful it was for me finally to let them go.

At eighteen, Tim left home to begin his tough training as a midshipman at Dartmouth Naval College. How well I remember putting him and his luggage into the train at Temple Meads Station in Bristol and saying goodbye. I told him, cheerily, that his dad and I had helped him get this far in his life, but from now on it was up to him. Months later, as I watched him in his passing-out parade at Dartmouth, upright and determined, I knew he was going to be all right.

Nic, on the other hand, had gone from school to university, where he read civil engineering. After two years of studying he was undecided about his future and needed a year away, working in Australia on his own to find out. When he came home he changed horses and found his niche in stockbroking. Now, a smart, determined young market-maker of twenty-four, he's very happy and independent.

During all those years both boys needed us, their parents, for help and support. But as I drive through Devon I have a strange feeling and realize I'm undergoing a difficult transformation, a change of roles. Now I desperately need the boys to support me.

I head on through the blazing midday sun, passing Exeter, and recall my happy years with the Devon County Agricultural Show. How I wish I had time to look up some of my old chums – but I know I haven't. So I press on, and eventually arrive at Stoke St Gregory in Somerset, where I've a lunch date with Derek Hector, a very dear friend.

He's a comfortable, plump countryman, born and bred in these parts some fifty years ago, and full of down-to-earth West Country sense and humour. He left his life on the farm many years ago to become a news cameraman for the BBC in Bristol. He first met John at boarding school when he was seven, but he and his wife, Audrey, have continued to be close friends to both of us since our divorce – something that most old friends have, sadly, found impossible to do.

Audrey is away, so we drive to the local for a real ploughman's lunch, where Derek reminds me of another crisis time in my life, twenty years ago.

He visited me then, in hospital, after my thyroidectomy and found me upset because of the operation scar across my neck. At that time I was a highly successful and much-travelled model, in great demand for fashion shows, photographic and television work. I realized immediately I came round from the operation that my blemish would severely restrict my work, even when it had healed. I was depressed, and thought I could never face a camera again or dance the catwalk.

Derek had told me to stop thinking about what I couldn't do and think about what I could do instead. His unique brand of humour soon had me laughing, and he set me thinking. He told me that BBC Radio Bristol was about to be launched and was looking for freelance contributors. He suggested I cut my teeth in radio broadcasting and that I concentrated, for the immediate future at least, on my voice and brain instead of my looks and movements.

As soon as I came out of hospital, I did just that. I was lucky enough to have Kate Adie, now a top BBC news reporter, as my boss and teacher. It was an exciting new challenge to be writing, reporting, editing and presenting. All good experience – in fact such valuable experience that I have called on it regularly throughout my career.

Today, Derek suggests I should again be looking forward, and not backwards with regret. And yet I have so much to look back on, both good and bad. I've led an interesting and varied life, the result of my own initiative and hard slog. And I've been blessed with many talents. I've tapped some of them already, but perhaps the time has come to expand others. Derek suggests I take up painting again, but this time seriously.

We finish lunch and drive on down to the family farm, aptly named 'The Willows'. On the marshy farmland grow the willows, or withies as they are called locally, which are used for traditional West Country basketmaking. I wander round the barns in the warm sunshine, as I have done on many occasions before. I watch some women sorting and stripping the willows once they have been removed from the boiling water which gives them their rich buff colour and lovely smell. In another barn, the craftsmen are bending 'and weaving the now supple stems, creating beautiful baskets and furniture. Outside, more men are busy making wattle fences with the bigger withies. In the corner of yet another barn, small sticks of willow are being cooked in huge ovens to become top-quality artist's charcoal.

Derek and his brother Nigel scoop up a bundle of assorted-sized charcoal for my inspection. Derek gives me some for inspiration and hopes I will soon put it to good use, sketching layouts for my new oil paintings. He reminds me that he's been waiting for an original thirty-one years – since we first met. I smile and tell him I'll see what I can do.

I leave my beloved West Country on a high note. What a tonic good friends are – but I'll be back this way again tomorrow. But as I drive past Bristol, my home for over forty years, and on towards London my spirits begin to sink. I breathe deeply, as Elizabeth told me to do on the phone yesterday. She, too, has been along this road, and she knew what emotions the past would evoke in me.

Peter and I arrive at the flat together. We're both very hot and tired. He is explosive, having had a bad couple of days in the office. In an attempt to explain his sudden changes of mood Mavis has told my secret to his staff, and he's very cross.

His attitude to me, too, is off-hand and hurtful. I try talking to him but he brushes me aside, seeming to ignore me.

I feel an intense anger mounting inside me, which I direct at Peter. I've tried to be so brave and cheerful over the past few weeks, and I don't feel I deserve this treatment. He snaps a reply to whatever I ask, and it's the straw that breaks the camel's back. The floodgates open. I'm furious, I'm tired and I've got cancer. Doesn't he care? Surely, if cancer is caused by stress, he's been the source of some of mine? I've taken on many of his problems and helped him when he was ill. I'm smouldering.

What about me and my future? I'm facing the possibility of no more work, and I haven't got a husband to lean on. My limited money won't last me long with my huge mortgage and high London expenses. I'm worrying my friends and family, and realize I stand to lose my financial, physical and – if I'm not careful – even my mental independence. I may become a burden to my family, and I face the immediate prospect of intense pain. But worse still, I'm about to lose some of my precious femininity. So who's the one with problems?

I tell Peter he can be so selfish on occasions. How would he like it if his balls were to be cut off? Then he really *would* have a problem. I've bloody well got cancer, and even with the operation I won't know for certain if I'll ever be rid of it.

Although it's early, I stomp off to bed and take a sleeping pill.

Friday, 24 June

Peter's very quiet this morning and leaves for the office before I get up. I haven't time to worry because I've got a lot to do. I'm off to the West Country again, down that damn motorway full of holiday traffic. Today I'm visiting my ex-husband, and I ring him to confirm before I leave.

But as I drive I start to feel sad about last night's outburst, and wonder if Peter will find it too difficult to cope. Poor man. He's been lumbered with more than he bargained for in his five years with me. . . .

We met through Mavis, whom I had known from Bristol where she had lived for many years, when I was looking for a London flat. She suggested I talked to her boss, Peter, who then recommended a new development in Battersea. He took me there before it was finished, and I found it difficult to envisage a nice home while looking at a building site. But he was a good salesman, I bought a flat – and he was right. For out of the mess and rubble rose a beautiful block of flats and small town houses.

It was many months before we met again – at a dinner party, arranged at his suggestion by Mavis. And it was several months again before he took me out for supper. Working on Breakfast Time *meant I had to have supper at 6.30 and be in bed by about 8.30 or 9, ready for the fiendishly early start. This was guaranteed to quash any romance in my life, and it was also difficult to find a restaurant with good food – let alone atmosphere – at that hour. However, over the next few months we saw more and more of each other.*

Peter's an attractive man, tall and slim with a shock of well-groomed grey hair which is rapidly turning white (although he disputes it). With dark brown, mischievous eyes and a seemingly permanent tan, he looks distinguished and older than his years. At first I took him to be my age but was shocked to find, a year later, that he was six years younger. Without knowing it, I had found myself a toyboy!

When his mind was on business he was sharp, quick and street-wise. But then, you have to be to survive in the property business. Socially he was good company, with his keen sense of humour and intense interest in the world of radio, television and entertainment. But, as I got to know him better, I realized he was very insecure. He had been divorced many years before, and since then had led a selfish and somewhat irresponsible existence, drinking heavily and apparently intent only on having a good time. Was I always so sensible? he asked me on our second date.

He could also be unpredictable, and would go off drinking and forget times and dates. During these sessions he could be very hurtful with his aggressive, chauvinistic attitude. I nearly finished our relationship after six months, but he was distraught and began to pull himself together.

I always felt there was someone very nice behind this odd façade, and caught little glimpses of him every now and again. But Peter was secretive and never talked openly about his family, upbringing, schooling, marriage or past relationships. Slowly I realized the extent of the hurt, and understood that a lot of covering up was going on. Carefully I revealed the very sensitive, kind person I now know so well – though, as with many people, the depth of his caring doesn't always show on the surface. His health had suffered, but gradually it returned to near normal, as did his pride and self-respect.

Within a year, he told me he wanted to spend the rest of his life with me. He sold his flat in London and we made a home together, buying a little place in Mudeford to get away from it all. Down in Dorset we found a life of tranquillity.

I arrive in Bristol and steel myself to visit John, with whom I shared twenty-five years of marriage. He still lives in the beautiful detached house that was our home for fifteen years. I feel apprehensive, but he greets me fondly and I'm pleased to find things look very much the same. Poppy, my old black cat, comes out of the kitchen to satisfy her curiosity and rubs up against me.

John produces a Pimm's – delicious, and the ideal drink for such a hot day. Then we sit down to lunch, which he has prepared superbly. He always was a better cook than me – well, a more inspired one, at least! We talk about the boys, and he speaks about their concern for me. He asks me if I'm going to marry Peter and I reply, simply and truthfully, that I haven't been asked. Then we chatter away about old friends and I catch up on all the business and local gossip.

As the time draws near for me to leave I ask John if I can have the face from the sundial by the pond in the garden. It was a birthday present to me from Jimmy, the husband of Dorothy, whom I'm off to visit next. It's very special, as he tooled it himself and gave it to me just before he died of cancer six years ago. Looking at it, I read: 'Time passes, but old friends remain.' Somewhat tearfully, I leave John waving sadly at the front gate. John's mother died of breast cancer in her fifties.

Dorothy is waiting for me – tall, elegant and beautifully poised. She used to run the best model agency in the West Country, and was my agent when I began modelling in earnest twenty-five or so years ago. Over the years she has become a mother figure to me, helping me through my fears and joys, professionally and personally. We are very close, and she is very concerned about me now.

She's more frail than I remember from my last visit, some months ago, and tells me she has been having trouble with her legs and balance. She has a keen sense of humour and amuses me with her account of a recent visit to hospital, to be checked over by the physiotherapists. They had asked her to walk barefoot for them. She did – elegantly up to the end of the room, where she executed a perfect model turn and returned with equal poise. They were amazed. Nobody had 'performed' like that before, let alone a lady of seventy-five. But unfortunately they couldn't diagnose her problem and she's cross at having occasionally to resort to a walking stick for support.

I'm glad to have seen her, and promise her a stay in Mudeford as soon as possible. She, in turn, is pleased to see that Jimmy's treasured present is in my safe possession.

I drive on to see my West Country surgeon, with whom I have an appointment. I have decided to seek his advice, and hope he will give me his blessing. He is sorry to have learnt from Mr Scott of the findings on the mammogram. However, he feels caution must be exercised. He advises me to have only the biopsy, and to wait two or three days for thorough tests to prove absolutely positively that I have cancer, before I make a decision to be operated upon. He advises me not to sign the consent form for a mastectomy. I should take time to consider the results of the biopsy and the proposed operation, and then make my own decision. This may prevent feelings of regret in years to come, wondering if it had all been necessary.

But surely, I ask, the mammogram has shown the problem to be there? He replies that he has not seen my mammogram and cannot therefore give me his final opinion. They can be deceptive, he adds. If he were convinced of the diagnosis, then he would approve of the treatment proposed.

I don't know what to think. I realize that surgeons, too, are human and can have different opinions. But what are we simple patients expected to do? How can we decide what's right or wrong, and what action has to be taken?

I drive on to my cousin Pauline's house nearby, and we discuss the events of my afternoon over a cup of tea. Pauline is pretty and petite, like both our mothers were. In her fifties, she has an enormous sense of enthusiasm and fun. We have grown close over the years, sharing joys and sorrows as we each reared our two children of similar ages. I begin to feel that perhaps I haven't got cancer after all. It could all be a mistake, and I feel quite optimistic. With her husband, Terry, Pauline and I cheerfully discuss the alternatives.

However, I've more travelling to do, so I get on the road and head south for Dorset. But alone in the car, as the miles go by, the confusion crowds in on me again. I'm hot and tired – I've done a lot of driving over the last two days. Close to despair, I cry most of the way to Mudeford.

Peter's already in bed. I close my eyes and hope it's just a bad dream, and that when I wake it will have gone away. But I can't sleep, and seeing me so troubled makes him most upset.

Saturday, 25 June

Peter and I lie in after a simply awful night. We try to make love, but can't.

We're quiet all day. I garden and prepare to be absent. Peter visits his mother and asks her not to call to see us this weekend, as she usually does. We want to be alone.

Late in the afternoon we take ourselves off for a long walk. After catching the ferry boat to the sandbank we walk, hand in hand, to Hengistbury Head and on along the miles of unspoilt beach. We feel apprehensive, and need one another's closeness, although we say little. We're both deep in our private thoughts.

Sunday, 26 June

We muddle through another quiet day. Pete and Marion invite us to a goodbye barbecue with a few other friends – they're off to Spain and we shan't see them for two months. Peter and I try to be bright and we enjoy ourselves, momentarily putting our troubles to one side. Only as we leave do I waver. I wish Marion and Pete *bon voyage*, but as they wish me good luck in return my eyes redden and Peter holds me tightly. The rest of the gathering think I've had a little too much to drink.

A sleeping pill is required tonight.

Monday, 27 June

Peter is amazing – we're both by nature early birds, but he's *always* sharp in the morning and today he's up and off at five o'clock. I snooze till 8.30.

I pack up house and cat and travel back to London at midday. Late this afternoon I have an appointment with Mr Scott and Mr Crosswell.

Just after five Peter joins me in the consulting room. He looks so handsome, if a little nervous, as he sits down beside me. It makes me even more determined to win this damn fight. I feel alert, with a list of questions, and if it's going to be, then I'm ready to get on with it. I've played this game of patience for long enough.

Mr Scott sets out his plans for the operation, and Mr Crosswell explains that, although he will be present, he will not necessarily operate. It will depend on what is found. Mr Crosswell tells us that from his experience he has found all women love their breasts and mourn their loss. But, having lost a breast, some women cannot bear the thought of reconstruction. Others feel mutilated and prefer immediate reconstruction if possible – I know that's what I would like. They set the date for next Saturday morning, and I'm to be admitted to hospital on Friday afternoon.

I take out my list of questions and start firing. Peter joins me, voicing his queries. We both wonder if this is all really necessary, and ask if it could be delayed in case the cancer might just go away. Both men are extremely patient, but finally tell us that we must eventually trust *someone's* judgement.

But I refer to recent newspaper reports on alternative methods of treating cancer, and to the many opinions I heard voiced on radio and television during European Cancer Week last May – ironically, the week before my terrible Friday the 13th. Neither surgeon, however, can recommend any of the alternative treatments. I, too, have not been convinced by the arguments I've read – I can imagine, for instance, that a radical change of diet might achieve something for cancer of the bowel, but surely not for breast cancer? And they put my mind at rest about the doubts raised by my West Country surgeon. My X-rays are quite unequivocal, and they explain that due to a regrettable oversight they were not sent to him. They are sure he would agree with their diagnosis if he had them in front of him.

Further to reassure me, they confirm that the mastectomy will only go ahead if the biopsy proves to be one hundred per cent positive. They tell me the consent form will be worded accordingly. If there is any doubt they will not continue, but consult me later to decide what, if any, further action should be taken. By coincidence, my West Country surgeon will be coming to the Royal Marsden on Friday, the day of my admission, and the three men have agreed to meet up to discuss my problems and review my mammograms.

This consoles both Peter and me and we feel satisfied. After an intimate supper in a nearby Italian restaurant we go home and sleep peacefully.

Tuesday, 28 June

At last the day has come for my long-awaited meeting with Elizabeth – someone who's experienced breast cancer herself and who can tell me what to expect.

But first a meeting of SOS, the Stars' Organization for Spastics, at their Regent's Park headquarters. As a new girl on the fund-raising committee I'm greeted kindly by the chairman, Noel Edmonds, and the charity's patron, the Countess of Arran. I find I already know many of the committee members, including broadcaster David Jacobs and comedienne Janet Brown. Noel embarrasses me by his official welcome: he comments how amazingly fit I look and how well I must be – sun-tanned, slim and agile. If only they knew I had cancer, I think. But then I remind myself that Mr Scott has told me I'm not ill. I listen carefully to their plans and am delighted to be able to help their worthy cause.

After the meeting and the buffet lunch that follows, I make my way to Elizabeth's flat in Fulham. I haven't seen her for five years, since the launch of my keep-fit book in the Orangery at Holland Park. . . .

She had been a guest of Christopher, my then agent. The press had been pointing their cameras at me for months. So, as arranged with Breakfast Time, *after my few words about the book the TV cameras were turned on them as I encouraged them to join me in a keep-fit session. It was spontaneous and hilarious, they were good sports and it resulted in some excellent pictures. The best one of all was of Christopher, who enthusiastically joined in and, whilst doing deep knee-bends, split the seat of his pants. He's never forgiven me!*

Today Elizabeth looks wonderful. She's a most attractive woman in her fifties, vibrant and amusing, with beautiful turquoise blue eyes. She settles me down in a comfortable chair whilst she makes coffee.

I feel an instant affinity with her. She's a comrade. Without hesitation I begin to question her, all my worries and pent-up emotions tumbling out with relief. Calmly and directly she answers my queries, assuring me that everything will be all right.

By coincidence, her surgeons were the same two as mine will be, although her circumstances were different. Like me, she had had a twenty-year history of lumps and had also undergone previous surgery. Finally, ten years ago, she had one mastectomy but was not offered reconstruction. Although she recovered well from the operation she was disturbed to have lost a breast and suffered psychologically. After many years she found a surgeon whom she could trust and who would reconstruct her. She says the reconstruction has enhanced her life, and she has now regained her lost confidence.

I can't help but drop my eyes to look at her chest. I hope she doesn't think I'm too rude. She has a beautiful figure and is exquisitely dressed in a fine silk blouse, through which I can see a pretty lace bra. If only I could see more.

After an hour or so, and with my questions answered, Elizabeth somewhat shyly asks if I'd like to see the result of the reconstruction. She takes me to the privacy of her bedroom and undoes her blouse. When she takes off her bra I see a nicely proportioned breast, complete with nipple, perfectly matching her other one. On closer examination I can make out the faint scars of the operation. I'm delighted. In fact, I'm over the moon at what I'm seeing. I hadn't expected anything so good.

Somewhat fearfully, I ask her if she thinks I'll look normal again after the operation, and wonder if I'll be able to enjoy sex and do all the sporty things I like doing. As she dresses, Elizabeth emphatically reassures me that I will be able to do everything again – even ski, swim and play tennis like she does. And, she adds, she'll be there to help me. I feel so relieved and happy, and she hugs me sympathetically and knowingly. She's been through so much but she's won her battle. This is just what I needed. She gives me the inspiration I've been looking for.

I feel on top of the world that evening as I drive with Peter to the Compleat Angler at Marlow in Buckinghamshire, where we meet Richard and Sue, our friends from Florida. They're in England for a short business trip. Sue confides in me that she may be pregnant, and I can see Richard listening proudly. I'm delighted for them. It's been a good day.

Wednesday, 29 June

Only three more days to go till the operation. Peter has taken the day off to play golf. Good therapy. To take my mind off things, I decide to shop in Oxford Street. I've a few odd bits and pieces to get, and if possible some orange shoes to wear at Henley tomorrow.

In Selfridge's, I go into the Holland and Barratt health shop and buy vitamin E capsules, which Elizabeth says she took to help the healing process. And I buy some vitamin B with C for good measure.

Suddenly I'm aware of a handsome, well-dressed young man of about thirty looking at me. He smiles. I don't think I know him, but in my business I meet so many people, so perhaps I do. He says hello and I nod. He's of Arab appearance, with a sweater slung fashionably around his shoulders.

I make my way up to the shoe department, where I browse through various shops within shops and stop to look at a likely shoe. A tap on my shoulder makes me jump, and as I turn the young man hands me a shoe for inspection. It's the Arab. Surprised, I thank him but say I know what I'm looking for and don't need his help. He replies that he only wants to help me and he'd love to spend some time talking to me. What a cheek. Politely, I say, 'No, thank you,' and walk quickly away.

Back in Oxford Street, I pop into another shoe shop – but the young man is there. I rush out and walk smartly on, hoping I've lost him. But as I try on a shoe in the next shop, I find him sitting alongside me. I tell him sharply to leave me alone.

I leave the shop in anger and decide to get on a bus to Knightsbridge to lose him. With relief I sit in the only vacant seat downstairs. The bus stops and starts in the heavy traffic all the way up Oxford Street, and at Marble Arch I move over to let my fellow passenger out.

As I stare out of the window at Hyde Park, looking beautiful in the sunshine, I become aware of a new arrival by my side. To my horror, it's the persistent young man. Fiercely now, I tell him once more to go away and defiantly look the other way out of the window. I breathe deeply to keep my cool.

Arriving in Knightsbridge I get off the bus, but he catches me up and walks alongside. I've had enough, but I'm too nervous to go home in case he follows me. He continues to pester me as I stride on and into Harrods. Up in the shoe department, I sit down and the assistant asks if I need help. I tell her I do – and ask her to call the store detective.

A little taken aback, she rings Security; but by the time the detective arrives the pest has fled. It did the trick. Perhaps I should have told him I'm not what I appear – I'm old and I've got cancer. That would surely have cooled his ardour. Alone, and in peace, I find and buy my orange shoes.

Back in the flat, I tell Peter the story. He tells me I'm too polite, and should have told the Arab to f—— off. We laugh. Relaxed and happy, we make love.

Thursday, 30 June

It's jolly good boating weather – just right for Henley. My orange and black silk suit from last year looks good with my new orange suede shoes. And my black silk hat looks smart with its band of material cut off from my shortened skirt. Peter looks cool in his blazer and flannels.

Clare and Peter meet us at the Remenham Club. Peter, who works in computers, is a member and rowed well for years until a recent back injury. His wife is a very old friend from Bristol. We were next-door neighbours as children, and a very mischievous pair of little girls at that. We were Brownies together, then Girl Guides and members of the same Methodist church and youth club – we've been friends, in fact, for thirty-eight years. We have no secrets from one another.

We all decide not to drink very much today. It's such a temptation at Henley; but we're conscious of not drinking and driving, and I'm pleased because I want to be as well as possible for my op. at the weekend. We stroll along the tow-path and sit in deckchairs at the water's edge. Boats with their eager crews skim along the water, while fashionable women in beautiful hats and handsome men in blazers and ridiculous caps wander around the lawns. One gentleman doffs his cap and compliments me on my appearance. I'm flattered. Lunch is in the elegant marquee – salmon salad and strawberries and cream, and just the occasional traditional Pimm's.

After lunch we saunter on down to the Leander Club. Here Clare proudly points out the many plaques on the staircase and around the walls, mementoes of her father's captaincy and rowing successes there years ago.

Tired but relaxed, we drive back to London . . . But when we arrive the flat looks a mess. Feathers and blood are all around the lounge. At the glass doors leading out on to the balcony lies a little bird, victim of Maggie. To my knowledge, it's the first bird she's ever caught. All that practice in Mudeford with the butterflies seems to have sharpened her skills, and this poor little thing has been snatched from the balcony. Maggie has become a hunter, and it's not a pretty sight.

It's been a lovely day, and cancer has been out of my mind altogether. As I lie in bed I feel there really is a good chance I may not have cancer, but I decide to put my trust entirely into the surgeons' hands. I hope the bird isn't a bad omen.

July

Friday, 1 July

It's an early start for Peter – up at five o'clock and off to Heathrow to catch a flight to Dublin. I visit Ian, who once again cuts and organizes my hair. It's important to me to know my hair looks good, because it will boost my morale.

I feel prepared as Elizabeth calls for me at 2.30. We arrive at the large private hospital in west London and I register. Some old West Country friends of mine, Jack and June, have sent a pretty arrangement of pink and white flowers with explicit instructions for them to be waiting for me on my arrival. What a kind thought – I couldn't have a nicer admittance.

Elizabeth and I make our way up to my small room, and the nurses begin their routine checks. A beautiful basket of orange lilies arrives from Nic, and an exquisite arrangement from Elizabeth herself. My friend Rosemary calls in with her new baby and brings a pretty bunch of flowers. We all sit down and chat happily.

It's very hot and I try to open a window, but the maintenance man has to be called to fix it with a special key. Obviously other people don't like fresh air as much as I do. Elizabeth tries the TV, but it's not working properly. Soon an electrician knocks on the door and comes in to fix it. As Rosemary leaves to take her hungry baby home there's another knock on the door. A tall, handsome, cheerful woman enters and tells me she's the gas lady. I'm amazed – I didn't know we needed anything more fixed. But she turns out to be my anaesthetist!

Elizabeth leaves me, now that I'm quiet and perfectly relaxed.

Mr Crosswell calls in quickly. He says he'll be standing by if he's required, and whatever happens he'll get me back more or less to normal. I tell him to forget about less and to make it more!

A huge basket full of potted plants arrive from my agent Annie and her angels. I'm touched. The door opens quietly, and as I look up from my magazine I see Christopher, his face hidden behind a basket of long-stemmed blue scabious, delicate pink roses and white orchids, smelling delicious. He hugs me, and we chat for an hour or so until a call from reception tells me that Peter's on his way up.

I ask reception to vet all my telephone calls and visitors from now on. I only want to see or speak to my few close friends and family, and I certainly don't want any snoopers. It's nine o'clock, and Peter's tired and a little flushed after his hectic trip, but I'm so glad he made it to see me settle in.

Mr Scott looks in, and together we decide on the wording of the consent form, which I sign. I want to be in charge of what happens to my body. Peter finds it difficult to leave me. We gently kiss each other goodbye. He hesitates at the door, but finally departs.

The night sister comes in swiftly to attend to me and asks me which of the handsome men is my husband. She's a comely black lady, kind and efficient, with a charming manner and smile. I bath and then climb into bed, but as I take the sleeping pill she offers me I feel choked with emotion. With strong conviction she tells me everything will be fine, and suggests I say a prayer to Him before I finally settle down. I do.

Saturday, 2 July

I tried to have a good night's sleep, but here I am at four o'clock in the morning, curtains and windows open and wide awake. I'm apprehensive, but not distraught. In fact, I'm impatient to get on. I wish I was the first of the operations of the day, but apparently I'm second of six. As I lie here, I look at all the beautiful flowers and feel very loved.

Soon enough my morning becomes busy. My blood is checked, and after a bath with a special pink anaesthetic rub I'm given two pills to make me more sleepy. I lie back and wait. Sister is very kind, and reassures me as I'm manhandled on to the trolley and taken down to the theatre. I've given many performances in my time, including two by Royal Command, but as I'm wheeled to theatre I vow this will be my finest yet . . .

When I wake up again, I feel a flash of the most excruciating pain I have ever felt in my life – and then, instantly it seems, blessed relief as painkillers are injected. The nurse tells me I've been in the theatre for four and a half hours. She says everything has been done, and slowly and happily I realize she means *everything*. I was so dreading waking up to find all they'd done was the biopsy – which would have been the case if there had been any doubt about the presence of cancer. I'd mustered all my strength for that moment of coming to after the operation, and I didn't think I could cope with enduring that experience twice. My mind at rest and my pain deadened, I drop back to sleep with relief.

I wake up feeling sick. I don't know if it's day or night. The nurse tells me Peter has been advised not to visit. I'm sure he must be worried. A wonderful arrangement of blue flowers is delivered. How appropriate – they're from my sailor boy, Tim.

Apparently it's night-time, but I can't sleep. I'm on my back and I usually sleep on my front. I'm a bit uncomfortable. As dawn comes, and the sun rises, I hear a rustle outside my window. I look more closely and see a pigeon feeding her babies in her nest in a small fir tree on the corner of my window ledge. How lovely and peaceful, right here in the centre of London. They amuse me for hours.

Sunday, 3 July

I feel very, very sick. The surgeons come in and cheerfully tell me what they've done, but I can't listen. I try to, but I'm sick in front of them. Peter calls, but I feel too ill to talk. He's most upset. The painkiller, Omnopon, is having a bad side-effect on me – I'm told it does that with some patients. Through the haze I'm aware of Elizabeth, who quietly holds my hand and reassures me. By the time I focus, she has gone, but the memory of her kindness lingers on throughout my incoherent day. My lunch is brought in, but I'm literally sick at the sight of it. Not a good day.

By evening I'm off the painkiller and life seems worth living again. I feel I've got my dignity back. Yes, there is pain, but I can take a tablet to deal with it if and when I need to. And yes, there is discomfort with all these tubes coming out of me everywhere. But I'm no longer being sick, and so I'm no longer being rolled over for an injection in my backside every time to try and prevent further vomiting. My self-respect is restored.

Peter anxiously comes back to see me and is relieved to find I'm a bit better. I try to be bright, but it's very difficult. He doesn't stay long, and when he's gone the nurse gives me some sleeping pills and I have a good night.

Monday, 4 July

I feel more comfortable and very positive this morning. Mr Crosswell calls at 7.30 and explains how he was able to reconstruct my breasts, as he'd outlined to me a few weeks ago. The prosthesis is a permanent one, I'm glad to hear, so he doesn't have to replace it with another at a later date. He assures me that everything is going to be fine. What a tonic he is – always cheerful and optimistic. Peter comes in on his way to work and is pleased to find me so happy. Mavis telephones to ask me if all went well. I decide I don't want any visitors today. I just want to concentrate on getting well quickly, which I know will be helped if I can rest.

I'd like to get out of bed and have a bath, but it's difficult. The top half of me is swathed in bandages, and coming out from either side under my arms are drainage tubes leading to bottles. The nurse and I put the bottles into polythene shopping bags so that I can carry them and be more mobile. But my right hand is attached to a saline drip which is held up high on a frame behind me. This contraption the obliging nurse wheels into the bathroom alongside me, and somehow, amidst a lot of laughter, I get into the bath.

It makes me feel much better, but I'm still nauseous. I take my mind off it by watching the Wimbledon men's finals on television. It's an excellent match, with Edberg beating Becker, and I'm glad it rained so hard over the weekend that the game had to be postponed. It's a bonus for me to enjoy today.

Somehow Christopher gets through the security and calls to see me. I show him my pigeon family, and he chuckles as he reminds me of a time when I stayed at his house in London during a hot spell a few summers ago.

Hearing a noise in my bedroom I woke in terror. Then I discovered that a pigeon had come into my room through the open doors from the balcony, where, unknown to me, it had its nest. It was busy pecking around my bed for tit-bits.

Christopher leaves as Peter arrives, looking more happy and relaxed. We chatter away quietly. As he leaves, Mr Scott arrives. He's pleased with the way things are going but apparently I'm anaemic, so he prescribes iron pills. If I keep up my good progress, he thinks I'll be able to go home on Wednesday. There's a challenge.

I finally settle down to sleep at 10.30, but I can hear a commotion in the corridor outside and then in the room next to mine. I ask the male nurse if the noise can be kept down, and he says he'll see what he can do. But it doesn't stop, the voices are loud and excitable, and doors keep opening and shutting as trays of coffee and people go in and out. It's now 11.15 and I'm beside myself. I call the nurse and remark that all the visitors should have gone by 9.30. Surely, he replies, I realize that this is a private hospital, not National Health? I'm speechless. There's no answer to that and, feeling miserable, I try to sleep as the noise next door continues. And to think I thought my health care scheme would guarantee me quiet and privacy – what an irony!

Tuesday, 5 July

It's four o'clock in the morning, and I'm wide awake. I've had little sleep and I need a painkiller.

Mr Crosswell calls at eight and removes the dressings from my chest. I see, for the first time, my small breasts which, although bruised and stitched, look in pretty good shape, even though I'm missing one nipple. He helps me into a surgical bra, which looks more like the liberty bodice I used to wear as a little girl. It flattens and constricts like a tight corset, but it holds the dressings and me in place. He tells me I will need to wear one all the time for three months.

On my own again, I feel quite human. I'm so thrilled with how I feel and look. I just want to cry – and I do, all alone with no one to see me. I've no self-pity – just an overwhelming sense of relief and joy that I've been given another chance in life. I vow I'll put it to good use, and then I feel at peace with myself.

The hospital administrator pops in to apologise for last night's incident. Apparently it is an Arab prince next door, with ten or so of his staff at his beck and call. She promises to move them or me before tonight.

The day is busy, with a constant flow of kind and thoughtful visitors. I'm very grateful. I look forward to a quick visit from Patsy, who phones to say she'll be passing the hospital on her way into town. Until her divorce many years ago she was married to Desmond Wilcox, the TV presenter, now the husband of Esther Rantzen. It's good to see her – she's so encouraging. Her life hasn't been easy, and we share a fighting spirit which helped us through our days together on *Breakfast Time*. Live TV is exciting but tough – your responses must be instant and perfect. It took a lot out of us both, especially at that hour of the day.

My cousin Pauline comes up from Bristol and is her usual cheerful and amusing self. Mr Scott keeps popping in and out. Peter calls to see me in the afternoon, bringing with him Richard, who's over from America.

Early in the evening Nic and my brother's eldest daughter, Lucy, travel up together from Bristol after work. Lucy is a pretty, dainty girl with a shock of sandy-coloured hair. I haven't seen her since she was fifteen and now, at twenty, she seems so mature. She's brought me a bunch of flowers and we sit and talk for an hour or so. John has given Nic a present for me. The heavy parcel contains four half-bottles of champagne. John has always known how to add sparkle and fizz to any occasion!

Nic's birthday is the week after next and I've shopped in advance for him. Together, Tim and I have bought him a lovely watercolour of sea and boats by Christopher Hollick. Peter has brought it in to the hospital, and now I give it to Nic as his early present. He's delighted. I've also bought a pair of sailing shoes for him, navy and green Docksiders, which I know he's wanted badly. He stands up in his smart City suit and puts them on, complete with their large labels still attached. As he does, Mr Scott comes in again, and we're all amused as Nic steps forward to shake his hand and trips up on the labels.

As the night sister settles me down, she assures me the Arabs have been moved. They had requested a larger room . . .

Wednesday, 6 July

A dreadful night. I find it difficult to sleep on my back, and I can't move much because of the drains in my sides. At least the drip has now been removed, so I do have a little more daytime mobility.

Mr Crosswell visits at the crack of dawn, and we arrange an appointment for me to see him next Monday at the Royal Marsden. He thinks I may go home today, but I still feel very sick even though they've changed my painkiller. I'm told it's the after-effects of the anaesthetic.

Peter rushes in on his way to work and keeps the taxi waiting. His visit is necessarily short, and I feel a bit depressed. I decide after breakfast to sleep it off.

I wake up feeling brighter and eat lunch for the first time since the op. Peter comes back in the afternoon and brings another Diana to visit me, the wife of Brian, one of his closest friends. She's a nurse, and she understands. They both cheer me up, as does the post when it arrives mid-afternoon. Many of my friends and relatives are thinking of me.

I try to read the papers and catch up with the news, but I find my eyes are a problem. I can't focus for long, and reading newsprint makes the sickness worse. I decide to stop the painkillers altogether – I'd rather have discomfort than nausea. But I can only reduce the nausea, not stop it altogether – the anaesthetic is in my body and will go on having this unpleasant effect on my eyes and stomach.

Peter calls back after work. He's worried about the office, and it seems likely there will be staff changes. Our spirits lift again with Tim's arrival at seven o'clock. He's exhausted, having driven up today from Dartmouth to Birmingham in time for Jill's graduation, and then down here to see me. Jill is now Dr Jill, and we're all delighted.

Mr Scott calls in to say he would like to take out my drains, but seeing Tim says he'll come back later. I'm a little embarrassed as I introduce them, since Peter has brought in some beer to refresh my tired son and my tiny room smells like a brewery. I hope he doesn't think badly of my boys – one on the booze and the other unsure on his feet!

I'm nervous when Mr Scott calls back at ten o'clock to remove the drains. By now I'm tired, and I'm not on painkillers any more. It's a very unpleasant business, but he does it with skill and the least possible discomfort. The bag lady is now debagged.

He is the most delightful man – sincere, thorough and amusing. Sitting back in the easy chair, he confirms my diagnosis from the pathologist's report. My cancer, being non-invasive, was confined to the breasts and therefore shouldn't reappear anywhere else in my body. I should be fit for at least another twenty years. He cautions me, however, to continue my vigilant watch for cancer, which, of course, could appear in another form – in my cervix, lungs or ovaries – just as it could in any other woman. He stresses again how lucky I have been that my cancer was not invasive, and suggests I thank the doctor at the Amarant Clinic for his astuteness.

He warns me I will feel very tired and reminds me I am likely to be short of energy even after the six or eight weeks it will take to convalesce. I must not lift anything heavy, or stretch my arms up too high. Finally, he confirms that I can go home tomorrow – I'm so pleased. We'll see each other again on Monday, with Mr Crosswell.

Thursday, 7 July

I don't care that I haven't slept well again. I'm just so excited at the prospect of going home. It's only five o'clock in the morning, and my pigeon mother is very busy with her babies. Quietly and carefully I get out of bed and pack my things. I take my flowers out of their vases and put them on the floor near the door. Cautiously I have a bath, and dress in my turquoise and pink tracksuit. I knew it would be excellent, and it covers my corset perfectly. After this I'm exhausted, so I sit back on the bed.

I know Peter will be getting up at 6.30, so I telephone him and ask him to pick me up when it's convenient. He could come before he goes to work, and we decide this will be an excellent way of avoiding the rush-hour traffic. And I'll be able to surprise Tim, who stayed in the flat last night and is still sound asleep.

The staff seem amazed at 7.45 when Peter arrives and begins loading up the car. They tell us we're too early for the administration to prepare my bill. We have to wait till eight o'clock.

On the way home, I feel every bump on the road. But soon we're back, I wake up Tim and we settle down together for a long breakfast. It's lovely to be home. As he leaves to return to Dartmouth, he kisses me goodbye and tells me he knew I'd come through all right. Roman Catholic Father Docherty, a chaplain at the college, has been saying prayers for me. Tim had to confide his worries in someone, he confesses. I'm very touched.

Alone, I slowly wander about the flat. My breasts are now very painful. They feel like two enormous boils about to burst. I'm so frustrated – I can't even do little things like pushing the plug into the electric kettle or washing or ironing, and making the bed is impossible. Pushing and pulling anything frightens me, and I'm not able to stretch and reach. I glance in the mirror – my hair looks awful. I feel cold, although the weather's warm, and decide to go to bed. But even a hot water bottle and the cat, gratefully curled up beside me, don't warm me up. I shiver and feel frightened. I get out of bed and try to close the window, but I'm beaten. It makes me angry.

I'm very glad when Peter returns home early. I suppose I'm a bit shocked as a result of the operation, and I've also got a sore throat. It's nature's barometer for me: I always get a sore throat when I'm down.

Cooking is not one of Peter's strong points, and I've wondered how we'll manage to eat. However, he surprises me tonight as we tuck into smoked salmon and a wonderful salad and celebrate with a bottle of wine. It all tastes so good.

We go to bed early, and I lie flat on my back like a corpse. Peter drops off to sleep immediately. But by now I've got a terrible headache and I lie awake thinking. Eventually I start crying.

Peter wakes and tries to cuddle me, but it's quite difficult and he's afraid he'll hurt me more. He tells me to be brave, and I do try. But we decide it will be best for both of us if I sleep in the spare room for the next few nights.

Friday, 8 July

Shall I take a sleeping pill, or not? I don't want it to become a habit. My father certainly didn't – but he had his own special way of doing it.

For nearly twenty years, from the time of my mother's death when he was fifty, he avoided doctors as much as possible. However, he was finally convinced that a hip operation could drastically improve his arthritis by helping him to stand more upright. Spondylitis, a condition of the spine, meant he was permanently bent over, and arthritis in his knee and ankles just added to the problem. But he was a spirited, strong-willed man and never complained.

Whilst he was in hospital receiving treatment and physiotherapy he was offered sleeping pills, because his lack of mobility meant he had difficulty in finding a comfortable position in which to sleep. On principle, he refused. His philosophy was to interfere with nature as little as possible. But, he said, if they insisted on him having something to make him sleep, he would like a tot of brandy each night. The staff were taken aback. But he assured them it would cost the National Health Service no more than the cost of the excess of drugs he'd seen around him. He was given his nightly tot.

I decide not to take a pill, but am uncomfortable and wake on and off throughout the night. I call out to Peter, but he doesn't hear me. So I fumble my way into the kitchen, hoping a hot drink may settle me down. Peter does then hear me and takes over, sending me back to bed. He brings in some Ovaltine and a little glass bell, which he tells me to ring if I need him again.

When I wake up, I find Peter has gone to the office to open his post. At nine o'clock he's back again and decides to wash my hair this morning. I kneel like a little girl at the side of the bath. It reminds me of my childhood and my mother. Sitting me in front of the mirror, he tries his hand at blow drying my hair. I tell him he has an excellent touch but his technique is somewhat lacking. I feel much better with clean, swingy hair. At ten he leaves for Winchester, for Holly's open day at school.

Perhaps I should take life more gently, I think when I'm alone once more. I've been so busy for years, and so many friends have told me to ease up and not take on quite as much. I begin to think my father was right when he told me, on my fortieth birthday, to cool it, to reorganize myself and not to let people take advantage of my good nature. Now, at forty-nine, I'm no chicken, although in my mind I feel young enough and my body responds well.

Yes, I will try and change my ways, to leave a little more time for relaxation. And that decision turns me to thoughts of my childhood which, despite my father's martinet approach to our upbringing, was often a carefree, happy time. No one has to tell children to make themselves relax.

My mother's sister Kathleen was my favourite aunt, as lenient as my father was strict. She encouraged me in my artistic pursuits and channelled my creative high spirits. There were three sisters and one brother. The eldest was Phyllis, next came Kathleen, then my mother, Maisy, and finally young Ken. Evelyn, a cousin who had been orphaned, also lived with them in Bristol. They were bright, happy children and were very close. But my mother's family was no stranger to tragedy.

Her father, my maternal grandpa Snell, died when he was quite young, leaving an invalid wife in a wheelchair. My mother, being the youngest of the girls and not so involved in her education at the time, looked after her – a task which she cheerfully undertook for some years until her mother died peacefully.

In the meantime Ken had become a successful accountant in Frome in Somerset, where he married a local girl, Jean. They had one son, my cousin Richard. But in his early thirties Ken died of heart failure, as a result of stress during and after the war. The three sisters were distraught at the loss of their young brother.

Phyllis, the eldest sister, was clever and went to university. In her thirties she married a farmer, Reg, from Berkeley in Somerset. But very soon afterwards she died from complications in childbirth, leaving a tiny baby, my cousin Mary, to be brought up by her father and his parents.

Reg moved back from his pretty cottage where the newly-weds had lived to the farm, where at first a full-time nanny was employed to look after Mary. When the nanny was on holiday, Aunt Kathleen, who was a deputy headmistress in Bristol, would move into the farmhouse with Pauline, her daughter, and me for company. Pauline and I had a whale of a time with Mary and our older cousin Richard, who lived just up the road.

Life on the farm was fun. Uncle Reg was a quiet, sensitive man and very kind. Being a single parent must have been difficult for him. The long hours demanded by the work on the farm left him little time to devote to his daughter. But he had the help of his mother, Kate, and his stepfather, Will.

Aunt Kate must have been very old at this time, perhaps in her seventies. I remember her as a wizened woman, bent and bony with a wax-coloured skin. She wore long, dark, old-fashioned country clothes and a bonnet. We found her very frightening.

Uncle Will, her second husband, was many years younger. With his large, bushy moustache, and sucking on his favourite pipe, he was a great character and we children all adored him. Both Reg and Will were tall, fine figures of men who dressed in traditional farming garb, with black leather boots and gaiters. Uncle Will was always full of fun and jokes, with Judy his loyal dog at his heels. He was very fond of us children and went out of his way to keep us happy. I followed him everywhere. He would lift me up on the back of the farm horse for rides, or take me with him when he went into the barns to hunt for the eggs laid by the free-range hens. He taught me how to milk a cow, and I would lie for hours in the straw in the loft above the rows of restless cows in their stalls, listening to the whooshing of milk into the metal pails.

The farm itself was beautiful, with a large, old farmhouse, yard, stables, barns and dairy. The churns of fresh milk were placed in the dairy to await collection, and we children would go in, fill a small jug with the warm, frothy liquid and drink it. It was nectar. Next to the airy, flagstoned dairy was the cool, dark area where the butter was made. One after the other we would laboriously turn the handle of the barrel of milk, which eventually gave us the most delicious fresh butter. The story of

Little Miss Muffet eating her curds and whey took on a whole new meaning.

The noise of the men's hobnailed boots on the flagstone floor still rings in my ears today, as does the sound of the door latches which I would open up if I wanted to go further into the house. The parlour was kept for Sundays, when it could be reached through the passage leading to the front door, which was not often used.

To go to bed meant standing on tiptoe and unlatching yet another creaky wooden door at the bottom of the stairs. The circular, dark staircase finally led to a passage and the bedroom which I shared with Pauline. The bed was a huge brass affair with a mattress which sent both of us girls into a giggling heap in the middle. There was no electricity. When we went to bed we took a candle in a traditional brass candlestick. I was terrified of the dark, and this nightly trek with candles flickering ghostly shadows around the passages and rooms did nothing to fend off my fears. Before finally settling down to sleep we would brush our teeth with salt and water.

Downstairs, in the large farmhouse kitchen, the main light came from an oil lamp which shed its glow over the men as they read their papers in front of the huge log fire. I well remember, on my first visit, being in disgrace and reprimanded – a rare thing on the farm – because I had fingered the pretty white lacy mantle of the lamp, which, of course, shattered.

The house smelt wonderful – good, fresh food and country smells. Upstairs, yet another latched door off the passage outside the bedrooms led to the cheese room, where the newly made cheeses were placed to mature alongside the apples and hams. The rind of a good English Cheddar can still to this day bring back my childhood memories.

The informality of life on the farm changed on Sundays, when we all dressed in our Sunday best. The men looked immaculate as we made our way to church, past the little churchyard where my Aunt Phyllis lay buried. The building itself remains one of the most lovely English churches I have ever seen. It was very small, and reached by a path which wove its way between ancient yew trees and crooked headstones. Inside, we gazed up at the beautiful dome, built like a miniature St Paul's Cathedral. As children we were all religiously aware, and took the lead from proud Uncle Will reading the lesson and singing the hymns with gusto. Sunday was always a day of rest – as much as the farm animals and their needs would allow.

There was little traffic in the narrow country lanes; we could paddle through fresh streams, picking watercress and catching minnows. In the spring we gathered frogspawn to take back home, and took cowslips and ragged robin to decorate the breakfast table. Later we crammed our mouths with autumn blackberries from the hedgerows and pinched apples and pears from the orchards.

In the summer, we made our way to the fields where the men were harvesting. We would play in the newly mown hay and then join the men in their lunch of bread, cheese, pickle and fruit, all washed down with home-made cider. At sunset we children sat high up aloft the load on the hay wagons as they made their way slowly but surely through the lanes back to the farm.

But despite the idyllic way of life my family seemed cursed in some way. Just a few years later my cousin Richard's mother, Jean, fell ill and died. Richard was left an orphan. He was sent away to boarding school, but his grandmother took charge of his upbringing and Uncle Reg helped all he could. Not long afterwards our holidays on the farm came to an end when my wonderful Aunt Kathleen suddenly died, only in her forties. My cousin Pauline found her mother dying in the bathroom from a cerebral haemorrhage – a terrible experience that I was to repeat in every detail all too soon.

Grief-stricken, my mother decided immediately that Pauline, now an orphan, must come to live with us. In a few short years my mother had lost her precious young brother and all her beloved sisters. In vain she tried to reason out why fate had dealt the family such a bitter blow. She suffered from migraines, which now grew more frequent, no doubt aggravated by emotional stress. Many days we would find *her alone in a darkened bedroom, sick with pain. But after a day she would become her cheerful self again. Two years later, when she died, we were all devastated.*

Now Uncle Reg and my father were the only two surviving parents, but we children were old enough to fend for ourselves. Anthony, Pauline and I were still at home, so we shared the housework and the cooking: we became domesticated overnight. Anthony had just completed his National Service in the Army, and Pauline was working as a secretary. Richard was away making the RAF his career, while Mary was at boarding school.

After two years, Pauline became engaged to Terry and left us to get married. I continued my friendship with John, whom I'd met at my cousin Patricia's twenty-first birthday party just before my mother died. After some years he asked my father's permission for us to get engaged. I was nineteen, and we were married six months later.

After my own wedding, my father announced his intention to remarry. I was delighted, having been concerned that he was now alone. His new wife, my 'Aunt Phyl', was a spinster who had been my mother's closest friend. In fact she had been a school chum of both my parents, for the three of them had been at grammar school together in Bristol. She was a very successful, hard-working career woman, intelligent and jovial – a handsome, immaculately dressed lady six foot tall. In their own way she and my father were happy. Aunt Phyl knew my father well enough of old to cope with his difficult temperament.

But very soon Aunt Phyl was found to have lung cancer. It was diagnosed too late for successful surgery, and she was to endure a slow and distressing death. Over the months I would go with my father to the hospital when he visited her, and we sadly watched her slip away. My father, now badly crippled with arthritis, was on his own again. He never complained of the pain, but it was a constant source of worry to me.

As the years passed, so the bond between us cousins has strengthened. As we've approached the magical age of fifty, we've shared a sense of awareness that we've passed the point at which so many of our parents' lives came to a sad and premature end. So we tend to live our lives to the full, packing in all we can each day, and are privately thankful for it. Every new day is special, and as I sit here, thinking of the past, I realize that for me it's never been quite so true as now.

There have been many occasions over the past five years when I've wished I could get off the band wagon. But in my profession it's impossible. If you're a big star perhaps you can take time off, but I'm small fry and there's always someone – in fact hundreds of them – waiting to hop into my shoes. I recall Frank Bough, the presenter on *Breakfast Time*, telling me that it's one thing to become successful and arrive, but it's another to stay there. What a vicious circle this way of life is. Money is required to keep you where you have got to, but that means long hours of mental and, for me, physical exhaustion. The trouble is, of course, that like most performers and communicators I love it – the euphoria of success which over-rides pre-performance nerves and agonies. I realize that, by having arrived, I have created a style and a way of life. Once there, I have a duty to behave and perform as my public think fit. But this costs money, effort, enthusiasm, family and friends – and I often wonder whether it is all worthwhile. But on the whole I wouldn't have it any other way.

My father would not be pleased to see the way I live now. He wanted me to have a 'proper' job and an orderly way of life, not one that hurtles me around the country, putting me into stressful, often bizarre, situations when I wear clothes that he would consider unseemly. He had died just before I shot to fame on BBC *Breakfast Time* in my figure-hugging green leotard and tights. I think all the fuss and press coverage would have upset him – but perhaps I'm wrong, and maybe he would have been quietly proud and amused. I'll never know.

He thoroughly disapproved of show-offs, and totally discouraged any display or performance from us children. In his strict way he forbade me to wear even the slightest trace of lipstick until I was seventeen, and I must have been the last of my friends to put my extra-long legs into stockings and leave my white school socks behind me. He disliked children growing up too quickly, and discouraged my interest in fashion and design. If I wanted to go out with friends I had to ask many days in advance, giving all the details. To stay with a friend, which he didn't allow often, meant letters from their parents and precise instructions on what I was and wasn't allowed to do.

He didn't go to the theatre or cinema, preferring to spend time at home with a good book. Years later, when even he had succumbed and bought a television set, he didn't watch it except for the news or a good play. Most entertainers were labelled and grouped. Girl vocalists were all called Moaning Minnies. I found it difficult to enthuse him with talk of my world, the world of showbusiness, without some sarcastic put-down.

His parents were equally strict and very proper indeed, but also kind and understanding. Sometimes, as a little girl, I came up from the country to stay with them in Bristol. In a drawer in the sideboard in the dining room Granny Dicker kept white triangular pencils, supplied by Brooks the launderers in Bristol, and she would produce one of these and a stack of paper for me to draw on. It kept me happy for hours. Although I was in awe of her, I loved my time with both her and Grandpa. Often we would ride in his big car, his pride and joy. After our customary rather formal high tea I would ask to be excused from the table and quietly slip into the kitchen. Here I would nervously sneak spoonful after spoonful of condensed milk from the tin. Such a treat. I thought Granny didn't know, but she had five other grandchildren and was well aware of my childish tricks.

She stood no nonsense, and bedtime was prompt. She would take me upstairs and, after my bath, kneel with me at the foot of the bed where we said our prayers together, Granny leading and me dutifully responding. When I grew tired I would crawl into the high bed and leave her alone on her knees in prayer.

Once tucked up in bed, I would lie and listen to the strange sounds of town – people's footsteps scurrying past, voices *and motor cars, none of which I heard in the quietness of my bedroom in the country. Even now sounds – as well as smells – can be strongly evocative, and when I'm away visiting I sometimes hear noises that for a moment take me back to my innocent, well-disciplined early childhood days.*

Granny and Grandpa lived their happy, ordered lives into their seventies. After Granny suffered a stroke Grandpa faithfully cared for her for years. Then one night he was taken ill and died, and Granny herself died later the same day.

I'm delighted to see a trusty confidante, Rosemary, who arrives with Alexander David, now just one month old. He's a handsome baby with big dark eyes like his mother's. She's brought lunch for us and a bottle of bubbly.

After they leave I realize my body hurts a lot, and I ring Mr Scott to tell him I'm not as brave as I thought I was and could he please prescribe me some painkillers. I decide to go back to bed for the rest of the afternoon, but not before ringing my agency to ask them to chase up my money owing.

The door bell rings and it's my fairy godmother, Elizabeth. She's been shopping and has brought me masses of fresh fruit, vegetables, cold chicken and salad. We're organized for a week.

Peter arrives home from Winchester, but the traffic has been awful and he's cross at having to go out again to get my painkillers. He's also upset that I'm obviously still in need of pain relief. But on his return he's in a better temper, and prepares supper.

I'm still in great discomfort, however, so I take myself back to bed. Lying down gives me some relief from the pulling sensations across my chest and under my arms. The whole area feels very inflamed and bruised, and I'm frightened of moving too much in case I pull the stitches and disturb the surgeons' work.

I sleep for a few hours, then wake at three and ring the bell. It works. Peter makes Ovaltine and gives me more painkillers. As I lie back, waiting for sleep to come again, I look at the crystal bell and smile wryly at the memory of the panto kids who gave it to me as a thank you present last year. I was most touched. They'd been lovely to work with – high-spirited but so well disciplined. None of us could have thought the bell would turn out to be so useful.

I was really sorry to have to cancel out of my part as Fairy Godmother in Bognor Regis this Christmas. Pantomime is such fun . . .

I made my panto debut with former Dr Who Colin Baker, Lorraine Chase and Derek Griffiths in Aladdin *at the Beck Theatre in Hayes, Middlesex. What an awful first night that proved to be! I played the Genie. Greenie Genie, of course – very athletic, a Genie on the Jog. There was a flash and a puff of smoke, and on I ran.*

Flashes are expensive, and for this reason not often used during rehearsals, so I wasn't quite sure what to expect. I stood anxiously in the wings and my cue came: Ebenazar rubbed his ring and called for his Genie. Flash! Terrified, I ran on stage through the smoke, opened my mouth to speak, choked, coughed, spluttered and turned scarlet. Derek, brilliant at improvising, shouted: 'Get thee to the pharmacy and return a fit Genie.' The audience laughed. I escaped off-stage, caught my breath and began again.

Last year I was in Cinderella *which must be the prettiest of all pantomimes, with ponies, spells, lizards, pumpkin and mice. My co-star was Nookie Bear, with Roger DeCourcey, and was he up to tricks! It's customary back-stage for cast and stage hands to spend time creating tricks to make other actors 'corpse' on stage. Roger suffers from flatulence and from time to time would quietly burp, which always made me giggle.*

As the Fairy Godmother, I was once again making my entrances with a flash. Unfortunately, one night my beautiful green fairy costume caught fire from the flash drop-out. I reacted quickly and averted a disaster, but burnt my arm a little. It became a bit of a joke, but as my script was entirely in rhyming couplets and we had a special performance for cast, staff and friends the night after, I got my own back. I changed the words. Flash! And on I went:

Though the front of house is thronging,
Back stage it's not quite nice.
There's a pair of ponies ponging,
And the stage is full of lizards and mice.

The back-stage crew keep flashing,
Puts me in a terrible whirl.
They set my dress on fire,
So I escaped on the stage with a twirl.

Oh yes, I keep my eyes open,
For surely this can't be right.
But I'm told things like this often happen,
So I hope it's all right on the night.

But that blasted bear keeps on belching,
Or maybe it's his friend?
Well, all in all, it's awful,
And it's driving me round the bend.

The Cinderella panto children loved it. During Aladdin I had soon found they were a breed apart, talented and disciplined. Along with others in the cast, they sent me a card as is customary on a first night. They had sensed my nervousness during rehearsals, so wished me luck, but told me not to be nervous because they would be there to help me through! They had nerves of steel, even at six or seven. Real little pros.

For my part in Aladdin, I was told I would wear the Genie costume from the wardrobe of the previous year's production, which is quite usual. But on seeing me in the flesh, the management realized I was too tall for the existing costume and would have to have another specially made. Natasha Kornilov, a theatrical costumier, measured me up and got to work. At the full dress rehearsal, the night before we opened, the cast was suddenly resplendent in full make-up and colourful costumes. But I was still in jeans – my costume wasn't finished.

As the rehearsal came to an end, the photographers arrived to take the official pictures. Natasha rushed in and I was whisked off, to reappear five minutes later in a figure-revealing costume. The body was bright green, cut like a leotard, but the legs were made of a flesh-coloured fabric and the whole thing made me look as if I had legs up to my armpits. Encrusted with glitter and sparkle, it was sensational.

David de Lacey, another theatrical costumier, was called in to design my Fairy Godmother costume for Cinderella. I was to be a traditional woodland fairy, but once again in shades of green. The eighteenth-century design started with a bottle-green top, with puff sleeves and a tightly fitted, low-cut boned bodice, which gave way to layer upon layer of flimsy material, cut with ragged edges which floated as I moved. The colours of the skirt graduated from bottle to bright lime green, while green leaves cascaded from the shoulders and decorated my crown and wand. Silver, gold and diamanté trimmed the dress and sparkled prettily in the lights. With a little sleight of hand from me a secret front fastening gave way and allowed me literally to step out of the dress, which was taken away by small fairies. It revealed my Green Goddess leotard and tights, in which I was able to put the children and audience through their paces.

Saturday, 9 July

It's been a very miserable, long night. At 5 a.m., feeling cold and sad and tearful, I leave the spare room and quietly climb back into Peter's bed. He cradles me in his arms as best he can, and we doze for another couple of hours.

It's one week since my operation. Hair washing restores my morale, and Peter sets about the laundry. We have a quiet, domestic day. I'm still very sore and my chest feels explosive. The three of us, Peter, Maggie and I, snuggle up together on the sofa and watch television. My eyes are still hurting too much to read for long.

I'm cheered by phone calls from the boys. They both assure me they'll ring whenever they can, just to check that I'm all right. I still feel pretty rotten, and I'm frustrated by all the simple things I can't do, but I feel instantly better knowing that Tim and Nic are thinking of me.

Sunday, 10 July

Yet another long night with little sleep. No wonder I feel a bit off today. I can't be bothered to have my hair washed. I just sit in the lounge and watch as Peter cleans the patio windows. Then he makes the beds, generally tidies up and gets on with cooking the lunch. He's doing an excellent job – he's even surprising himself.

My boobs still feel as if they're going to explode. Lifting my arms up is painful, and crossing them in front of my chest excruciating. I can't put anything on over my head, so a shirt or a jacket, or anything with a front opening, is the easiest thing to wear. I wonder if everything is all right. Maybe I've got an abscess. Or could it be that not all the cancer has been removed, and now there's some activity? Perhaps there's a rejection of the silicone? I have my daily bath, but can't see anything because I mustn't disturb the dressings. I feel very sore and nervous, and I'm glad I'm going to see the surgeons tomorrow.

Monday, 11 July

The painkillers are working and I sleep through till 3 a.m. That's an improvement. I ring the bell for the night service and settle back again. At six o'clock I feel wide awake, better and optimistic. Peter washes my hair and dries it quickly before he goes to work. It's frustrating not to be able to cope on my own, but reaching up still hurts.

My hair hasn't always been this colour. In fact it's naturally dark with a slight chestnut glint which I used to highlight with henna. But after a fashion show ten years ago it was pointed out to me that the colour was distorted by the stage lighting and looked too burgundy. I asked my West Country hairdresser to do something about it, but when he came to wash off the substance my hair had turned the colour of a ginger biscuit! He explained that a chemical reaction did sometimes happen, and that he could put it right, but he advised me to wait a week in order to keep my hair in good condition.

Two days later, however, I auditioned for the job of Continuity Announcer for HTV in Bristol, and got it. They had accepted me not only for the way I worked but also for how I looked, and I could hardly reappear looking very different. So I stayed with the colour, which my hairdresser toned down a bit and which subsequently lightened naturally in the sunshine as the months went by.

From that job, I was asked to join the ITV network magazine programme Here Today, which I did successfully for several years. BBC Breakfast Time saw me on it and invited me to join them. By now I was established, and the public at large knew me as a blonde. There was no going back.

Patti, a young Filipino, arrives at nine o'clock to help me with the chores. She shares a house with my cleaner, Virginia. Patti is in between jobs, and has volunteered to come each morning for several hours. She's tiny and doll-like, with shining dark bobbed hair and a flashing smile. But she's very capable and she takes charge immediately.

Elizabeth arrives at midday to take me to the Royal Marsden. I swallow a painkiller, because I know the dressings will have to be removed and some of the stitches taken out.

A tall, sun-tanned man is standing in the corridor as we walk down to the waiting room. He watches us pass by and both Elizabeth and I smile at each other, surprised to see a man here but delighted he's such a handsome one.

I'm called almost immediately. To my embarrassment I find

the man in the room along with the two surgeons. I'm introduced to him. He is a cancer surgeon over from Greece, and he was in the theatre with them during my operation. And to think I'd slept through the entire performance! I blush.

My dressings are removed, but they decide to leave the stitches for the time being. 'Super job,' says Mr Scott, smiling at me. Both surgeons inspect my breasts and smile at each other with satisfaction. The Greek god smiles. Sister is called in and she smiles too. It's infectious and I join in. Everyone's pleased with what they see. Mr Scott turns to the Greek god and, pointing at me, says, 'Super.' Everyone laughs as they explain to me that only minutes before the Greek god had asked for a translation of Mr Scott's well-used word, 'super'.

At home I show Elizabeth my breasts. She's amused as I drum my feet on the floor in childish excitement. I'm so happy and so relieved that everyone feels the operation has been a success. She leaves me and I run a bath. But without Peter here the taps are too stiff and awkward for me to turn, and I nearly have a disaster. I must call the plumber.

As instructed, I wash all over and then shower off. Carefully and slowly I ease myself out of the bath and catch sight of my reflection in the mirror. I stand in front of the mirror and take a long, hard look at myself. It's unbelievable. If I squint a bit, the image becomes blurred and I don't notice the extensive bruising, the cuts and the stitches. I'm whole. To my eyes today, I look and feel like Venus arising from the waters.

Immediately I feel much better and think of the future. I look quite normal. Nobody will know. I'll be able to wear all the clothes I want to. Swimwear, evening dresses and even my new white teddy, the lacy creation I treated myself to before I went into hospital.

OK. So I've lost a lot of feeling in my breasts and one nipple too – so what? I've got my life and my health. It's a small price to pay. I know now that I made the right decision when I chose to be operated upon. To go through life waiting for changes to occur in the cancer would have made me a nervous wreck. As it is, I can put it behind me and get on with living.

Tuesday, 12 July

I'm paying for my break-out yesterday, and feel very uncomfortable indeed. It's been such a long time since I woke up feeling refreshed and looking forward to a new day. Oh, please God, let me feel like that again soon.

Harry, the plumber, arrives and sees to the bath taps. Patti gets on with her work and keeps me company. During the afternoon Elizabeth comes to see me, loaded down with a home-made chicken stew and egg custard – very nutritious. Peter's pleased to see everything is in order when he returns and gratefully tucks into Elizabeth's goodies, relieved he's off-duty cook tonight.

As I prepare for bed, I decide to show Peter my breasts. I can sense his apprehension. I feel embarrassed as I carefully take off the corset and look down. But I'm tired and a bit low, and to me look disfigured and ugly. I can only see the cuts, the stitches and the bruising, and I feel the pain. Peter's kind, says he thinks I look all right, and assures me he'd say so if I didn't. He knows me well enough to understand I want the truth, not soft words and flattery. But I'm still not convinced.

Wednesday, 13 July

It's two months today since I was told I had cancer. My body really knows now that it's had a major operation, and I decide to stay in bed resting.

Peter returns from the office at lunch-time and gives me a lift to the hospital, where I'm to have the stitches out. Travelling isn't comfortable. I'm anxious and feel every jolt, turn and bump of the journey. My chest is bursting – I feel I could feed six babies.

But at the hospital I'm told not to worry. Mr Crosswell looks at my breasts but decides again not to disturb the stitches. He gives me another corset, some dressings and some calendula cream. It's made from marigolds, and I have to rub it into my breasts every day to massage them and make the skin soft.

Exhausted from my trip out, I have an afternoon sleep. Lea, a young friend from Bristol, arrives in the evening. She's heard I'm not well. I don't give her any details, and consequently she stays a little longer than she would have done had she known. I feel shattered when she leaves. But it was kind of her to come and I enjoyed her youthful company. I need a sleeping pill *and* a painkiller tonight.

Thursday, 14 July

I've slept a little better, and wake up feeling great. I decide not to take any pills for the pain today. I phone the doctor at the Amarant Clinic to thank him for being so astute in his observations back in April. He tells me again how fortunate I was.

At lunch-time Jean Moss an old friend, calls to see me. She's a brave lady with problems of her own. Don her husband, was a colleague of mine at HTV West and BBC Radio Bristol. He and Jean have brought up their severely handicapped daughter Susannah, now twenty-one, at home. They never complain and are always cheerful. I feel humble, and realize my troubles are few in comparison with theirs.

The proofs of *Look Good, Feel Great* have arrived for me to check, but I don't really feel like doing them. By 9 p.m. I'm exhausted. It's a relief to get into bed, and I begin to realize my recovery is going to take a long time. I am becoming aware of the seriousness and implications of cancer. I worry that the disease may recur if even small amounts of affected tissue have not been removed.

Friday, 15 July

I wake up at 3.30 feeling awful, then drowse till five. I crawl into Peter's bed for comfort. He chivvies me on and gets my spirits up, but I'm tearful.

At six o'clock he washes my hair and makes me have a bath while he's still around to keep an eye on me. The taps are easy now, and therefore safe for me to use, but I'm still not as nimble as I'd like to be. Everything takes that little bit more time. I shower off my breasts, dry them with a towel and finish them with a hair dryer – perfect dryness is essential. I ladle on the marigold cream and massage the skin, which is very hard, lumpy, bruised and painful. I have to take care not to pull the stitches. Then I replace the dressings and the corset.

Even though it hurts, having done all this makes me feel more perky. I decide to be more sensible today and spend the morning with my feet up. I can read those proofs.

The flat's full this morning. Harry, the plumber, has come back to do a few of the odd jobs I've been meaning to see to for a long time. Patti brings me roses, freshly picked from her garden. She's always smiling and I ask her what makes her so happy. She tells me she's a devout Catholic and she works hard. She loves her family, who are less fortunate than herself, and like many Filipinos in this country she sends money home whenever she can.

She's being such a help to me in her quiet, efficient way. I hadn't realized how short of energy I'd be or how many simple everyday tasks I would be unable to do for a few weeks. As she finishes her work she calls out goodbye. But she comes back in, walks across to the sofa and hugs me. She tells me she knows I'm being brave, but adds that she and Virginia have been saying prayers for me every day. I feel touched, and the roses smell even sweeter. I know Elizabeth is a practising Roman Catholic too, and am thankful of the support Tim has received from the Catholic chaplain at Dartmouth. I've always had firm religious convictions myself. I've been a member of both the Methodist Church and the Church of England in my time, but I know, especially at a time like this, that it doesn't matter what you call it – it's all faith.

I started out baptised into the Church of England, and in the days of my early childhood we always went to church on

Sundays. Later, when we moved to Bristol, our next door neigh-bours were fervent Methodists. Influenced by their daughter, my friend Clare, I too became a staunch Methodist, attending chapel and Sunday school and even taking the pledge. When my mother died I felt the true depth of Methodist kindness. With-out their help and care I would have been in the blackest despair.

When John came into my life he accompanied me to chapel – less out of religious zeal, perhaps, than because he wanted a chance to be alone with me. Given my strict father, this was the only way to do it! We were intending to get married in my local Methodist chapel, but this presented problems because John was Church of England. Eventually the minister suggested a compromise – he would marry us if I promised not to touch alcohol. But this seemed like hypocrisy to me: I was marrying into one of the big Bristol wine-shipping families, and it was unlikely I would be able to keep my side of the bargain. So I went back to my Church of England roots, sought instruction, and was eventually confirmed and married by an Anglican clergyman.

Elizabeth phones to tell me of a centre outside London which counsels people who've just had mastectomies. We decide we must visit them soon. When she had her operation Elizabeth had a vision of looking like an Amazon. These extraordinary mythological warrior women used to cut off one breast in order to use an archer's bow more skilfully.

It's strange how the mind plays tricks. I've already seen myself as physically reborn, like the goddess Venus. I *will* be strong and athletic again, although I'll never be quite the same. I watch others keeping fit on TV and wonder if I'll be left with some disability. I've observed people who have been afflicted in this way, and some of them have become a little bitter. I must guard against this, because I've always had a slightly jealous nature.

But on the other hand good can so often come out of the bad things in life. I know that part of my own character – my sympathetic nature, my love of people and the pleasure

I get from motivating and caring for the less fortunate –
stems from the loss of my mother, the most important and
tragic experience in my life. It formed an abrupt ending to my
childhood. Tears can still well up when I think of my mother,
her two sisters and brother all dying between the ages of thirty
and forty-seven. At least, at forty-nine, I still have my life. And,
my God, I want it – I've so much yet to do.

*My father chose to take early retirement a few years before
my mother's sudden death. He invested in a small shop selling
sweets, tobacco, toys and a few basic groceries. The idea had
been warmly welcomed by my mother, who saw it as a chance
to fulfil herself at last. She had never before had the opportunity
to work, but now she and my father could do this together. She
would run it from behind the counter, for she loved meeting
people and had a patient and understanding manner. My father
would tend to the business side of things, keeping the books
and dealing with stock control and orders.*

*It was a good plan, but after her death it backfired and the
shop became a trap for him. He was tied to long hours, and
didn't like the idea of taking on a stranger in place of my
mother. But he wasn't good at dealing with customers, and
he wasn't really cut out to run a small shop. By this time his
arthritis, which was later to cripple him, had set in. He found
it difficult to cope or to have time off, and over the years his
health deteriorated.*

*By now I was working in a large department store in Bristol.
Having completed one of my two years of commercial training,
and wanting some pocket money, I had found a holiday job.
It entailed a bit of everything – working behind the counter,
running errands and rearranging the stock – but best of all
helping to dress the windows. I was quick and eager to learn,
and loved the busy atmosphere. But my father needed a break,
so I finished at the store and ran the shop for him whilst he took
a holiday. After that I was due to return to college, though I
knew I didn't want to go back. I was then approached by
the store's personnel officer, who, perhaps impressed by my*

enthusiasm and ability to get on with people, asked me if I would like to join her and train to be a personnel officer.

When I told my father on his return, he was very angry. If I did so, he said, he would wash his hands of helping me with my career. What he really wanted, I discovered later, was for me to complete my commercial course and become secretary to a solicitor friend of his. I can understand now why, with my mother dead, he felt this urge to be over-protective to his daughter and didn't want me to go out into the world. But I still don't agree with it. In any case I had made up my mind. The next week I took up the offer and began work in earnest. Despite his attitude, however, my father still needed my support, and I gave it. Over the next three or four years, for part of my annual holiday from the store I returned to the shop whilst he took a much-needed break.

Now, at eighteen, the height which had once been such an embarrassment, and which I then turned to use on the athletics track and the sports field, suddenly became an advantage again. The store was to hold a fashion show, to launch its arrival in a new shopping precinct. By now the fashion buyers had become my friends, and suggested that, with my height and long legs, I would make an excellent model. After some persuasion I agreed to take part, and nervously tripped the catwalk for the first time. I loved the experience, and it whetted my appetite. Dorothy, who was later to become my agent, was the compere that evening and her 'girls' the professional models who helped me take my first steps.

This was to be the start of a lifetime of fashion modelling. Some months later a photographer friend asked me to appear as a young housewife in an advertisement for the South West Electricity Board. It set me en route for a successful career as a photographic model as well. It wasn't all as glamorous as it sounds, mind you – I used to do mail-order catalogues, and it was hard work trying to look seductive in long granny bloomers!

During the early years of my marriage I worked part-time, fitting the work in around my small children but rarely taking a job in their school holidays. Occasionally, if a small child was required, one of the boys would appear with me, oblivious to the fact that we were 'working'. As they grew up and started to lead busy lives of their own, with school and sporting activities, I gradually extended my working life. There was always more work than I could take on, and every day was different. I tried to divide my time between family and career, and most of the time it worked well. A group of several young mums, similarly minded, co-operated with each other and we were able to strike a happy balance.

As a model, I learnt to perform in the most unusual places. One memorable show was held in the elegant surroundings of the Pump Rooms in Cheltenham. Back-stage, things were less elegant. Our changing rooms that day were the large kitchens, and rehearsals were made more fraught when we sprang a leak – the plumbing, that is, not the models! Workmen were called to the rescue and seemed quite happy as our entrances, exits and hectic changing continued around them. However, one plumber was heard to mutter to his mate, 'Cor, I thought my missus were quite normal till I'd seen this lot.' What he had seen was a collection of healthy young ladies full of life.

But we models weren't always what we seemed, and we learnt to be versatile not just about the venues we worked in. A carefully unwound roll of cotton wool would turn a size twelve into a (literally) well-padded fourteen or sixteen. We even modelled underwear like this, and the audience never suspected. Those were the days, too, when a model's hair was never quite good enough on its own, and we stuck on a whole assortment of false hairpieces. No wonder that plumber got a shock!

Over the years, until the birth of the Green Goddess, I danced my way down the catwalks of major shows in this country and abroad. It led me on to train young models and to choreograph and present spectacular fashion shows in London and around Britain.

The photographic work resulted in television commercials, of *which I made hundreds for local stations. Before long I was cast in some of the major national TV commercials, including Oil of Ulay, Avon cosmetics and Cadbury's Marvel. As I became more popular I turned my skills and my voice to video presentation and radio commercials.*

They were hectic years, and I often travelled to four or five different venues a week. But it was this variety, so far removed from the steady, safe job that my father had been so determined I should have, that appealed to me.

Yet as I grew up and experienced motherhood, I started to see him in a different light. It can't have been easy for him suddenly to find himself overnight both mother and father to my brother, cousin Pauline and myself. He had always been dictatorial, of course, and now he became, if anything, even more so. I can see now that this was the only way he knew to control us children and bring us up to keep out of trouble. As the years went by, he and I became closer and I began to understand his eccentricities.

But he must have had a way with the ladies, for some years after Aunt Phyl's sad death he married for the third time. His new wife was a spinster and retired headmistress. She had been our neighbour, and as children we had been somewhat afraid of her. She looked after my father, which can't have been easy, until his death seven years ago.

His funeral was upsetting. My stepmother had requested no announcements and no flowers, and the ceremony at the crematorium was to be the simplest possible. On entering the Chapel of Rest she slipped into the back pew, and I felt it right to support her. A female friend of hers, my brother and his wife attended, along with John and the boys, and my father's elderly sister. My father's coffin was brought in, bearing on top a small red rose, a farewell token of my love. As soon as the simple ceremony was finished, my stepmother departed with her friend and we went our separate ways.

Judy, an old chum of mine from HTV in Bristol, calls to see me during the afternoon. She's good company, a fellow Gemini and very typical. She's been so loyal, sending cards daily to cheer me up and make me laugh.

In 1979 she was production assistant to my producer, Alex Kirby, when I was doing the networked afternoon magazine programme Here Today. *They were fun times, and I was particularly involved each week presenting keep-fit, diet and fashion. It was on this programme that the Green Goddess was born.*

The set for the programme was beige, yellow and green – very pretty and spring-like. Alex suggested that my clothing should blend in with the scheme, so I took myself off to London and bought a yellow leotard and tights from the Dance Centre in Covent Garden. It was rather avant-garde, for in the late seventies the keep-fit movement was still in its infancy. I tested the outfit under the studio lights – unfortunately I looked like a huge prancing canary. Next I tried what I thought was a classy beige leotard and tights – but to my horror I looked nude on screen! We were left with the green – an awful shade of lime – but despite my moans Alex said it would have to do.

But the shiny green suit looked sensational on set, and I soon acquired nicknames from the crew, many of whom I'd worked with at HTV for over ten years. They called me the Jolly Green Giant, the Incredible Hulk and, more kindly, the Green Goddess. The name was not used officially at HTV, only in good-humoured jest.

The programme was a success and we had a two-year run. During the second year the BBC were putting together ideas for their new morning show. They saw me on Here Today *in my green outfit, and invited me to become part of their team to launch* Breakfast Time. *My nickname of Green Goddess soon became well known, and the press loved it. Funnily enough, the outside broadcast crew at the Beeb rechristened me with their own favourite name, Kermit. I was certainly stuck with green. Fortunately it has always been my favourite colour, though until the birth of the Green Goddess I had usually worn more subtle shades. I've been called all sorts of names by the press, but the most memorable came from Jean Rook of the* Daily Express, *who on my first appearance on* Breakfast Time *likened me to a manic green caterpillar. Even in 1988 a journalist described my beautiful green Fairy Godmother's dress in* Cinderella – *most unfairly, I thought – as a creation resembling a bright green shredded lettuce.*

I did have some funny moments on Breakfast Time – *like the time we started a live broadcast from Swindon Fire Station with me sliding down the pole. But it was only with a little help from my friends the firemen. I suffer desperately from vertigo, and no one could persuade me to jump across the gaping hole in the middle of the upstairs muster room, grab the pole and slide down. The gallant firemen, no doubt used to chickens like me, placed a plank across the hole. Ten minutes before transmission, they encouraged me to edge my way across. I clung to the pole like a koala bear, and then the plank was whisked out of sight. It was a long time to wait, but on cue I whizzed down into vision, touched base and happily continued with the programme. The firemen swiftly followed me down the pole and grinned broadly as I put them through their paces.*

On another occasion – a grey, wet, miserable morning – I started at dawn in Plymouth on the deck of HMS Brazen. The entire ship's company had been ordered by their captain (a keep-fit nut) to be present. I was piped aboard, an honour until then reserved only for the Queen. Then I swung into action, and soon everyone on the deck was moving.

One young officer, trying to hide behind the others, caught my eye – to my astonishment I realized it was my son Tim. Apparently the secret had got out that the Green Goddess was his mum, and unfortunately for him his ship had come into harbour the night before. To his surprise he was ordered out of his bunk at some unearthly hour – I'm glad I wasn't there to hear what he said when he learnt just what for.

I have a video of that morning's programme, and it always

makes me chuckle. The deck was very wet, and the sailors were in full uniform. As I instructed them to lie on the deck their faces were a picture. You didn't have to be able to lip-read to understand what they said. However, it was a proud time for me.

I didn't enjoy myself quite so much with the Army in Aberdeen. Four programmes for that week had gone well, and the fifth was to be pre-recorded on the assault course. It was one of the toughest the Army had, I was later told, and used for training for the Falklands.

Complete in Army uniform and new boots, I was part of a four-person team competing at speed up and over a twelve-foot granite wall, along planks, and under and through obstacles such as smoke and water. I was pushed, pulled and shoved. Finally, I clambered up and on to the high scramble nets, where I froze. The vertigo got me again. The instructor shouted, the lads shouted and I shouted. It's amazing what language comes forth when you're pushed to your limits! The instructor, realizing the predicament, said, 'Get yer 'ands on 'er ass, lads, an roll 'er fast,' and they did. I fell down the last rope and stood shaking with terror.

Patsy, my producer, said in her sweet way that it was very good, but unfortunately there had been a technical error and I had to do it 'one more time please'. My body was tense with anger and fear. As a result I landed badly at the simple water jump, broke a bone in my heel and landed up in an Aberdeen hospital.

Another occasion found me nearer home at Battersea Heliport, off to visit the Army Air Corps at Middle Wallop in Hampshire. I was to be filmed at the time, and thought the Green Goddess would be living up to her colour that morning. But things went well.

Ten minutes later, however, we landed out in the country and I was transferred to another chopper. Only then did it dawn on me that I'd been tricked, and minutes later I was in the lead helicopter of the Eagle Display Team, in the middle of a display of aeronautics. In formation, we did victory rolls and other manoeuvres with split-second timing, cutting our engines – in fact, the lot. I should have been terrified, but it proved to be one of my most exciting experiences on the programme.

Working on Breakfast Time meant I was out of sync with others. Lunch-time was elevenish, supper-time sixish, bed-time 8.30 to 9 p.m. One snowy winter's night found me in bed in a Glasgow hotel, fast asleep, ready for an early morning start. I was woken by a persistent alarm – not mine but the fire alarm. Totally disorientated, I thought through my priorities. Handbag, briefcase, raincoat, boots. It was freezing outside as people gathered and the firemen went about their business. I collected my senses and became aware that everyone else was fully clothed and very jolly – some even had drinks in their hands. I, on the other hand, had no make-up on and, worse still, I was wearing only my burberry, which had an open split at the back right up to the waist. Everyone told me the alarm was new and over-sensitive, and that this often happened. I was soon recognized and, panic over, invited back to the bar for a drink. What was the bar doing, open at this time of night? To my embarrassment I then realized it was only ten o'clock at night, and not the wee small hours. I declined their kind offer and in record time returned to the safety of my room.

Another embarrassing but amusing moment resulted from a lovely hot summer week when I took members of the Upper Crust Roehampton Tennis Club, in London, through their paces. The week had gone well, and on the Friday I decided to do leg exercises on the court. In rows, either side of the net, everyone bounced up and down doing deep knee-bends in time to the music. After I had wound up the session I caught my train back to Bristol.

Esther Ranzten rang me at lunch-time: 'We want to have you on the programme this Sunday.' I asked her what for. 'Don't worry,' she replied. 'You've already done your bit this morning on Breakfast Time, and we've got the film.' Somewhat confused, my family and I watched That's Life on Sunday evening. As Esther introduced the item she told viewers to 'watch our Green Goddess, elegant as ever, but listen carefully to what she has to say'. Watching apprehensively, I saw my class bouncing up and down and then heard, to my horror, what had caused the humour. I had wound up the session by saying, 'Well, that's all from Roehampton Club this week, but as you can see, it's not only balls bouncing on the courts this morning, it's members too.'

Once the BBC sent me to the Norwegian fiords aboard a Russian cruise ship full of Saga holidaymakers. I co-opted the crew to teach us Russian dances, and coerced several well-known English footballers, guests aboard, to let us into their training techniques. Even on the flight home we recorded chair exercises for weary airline passengers. We didn't miss a trick, and were always on the look-out for unusual and bizarre situations for me to take on.

It caught the attention of the world press, and several American TV stations, including NBC and CBS, sent reporters to cover my activities. They came with us as I put Jersey potato farmers through back exercises in their clifftop fields at the crack of dawn, and to a knicker factory where I put workers through exercises for the bottom. Italy, France and Australia showed great interest, and I even made the front cover of a Russian magazine. It showed me working out with early morning commuters, complete with umbrellas, on Waterloo Station.

The gendarmes on the Champs-Elysées didn't know what had hit them when I did exercises with them. I had been sent to Paris to do a live broadcast for Breakfast Time on the morning that the rival ITV station first went on air with TV-am. I was there not because of my editor Ron Neil's love of fashion, but because he knew I had quite a following by now. The Green Goddess had caught the public's attention, and the programme needed to keep its viewers. The BBC had beaten ITV in the race to get early morning television on air, which had been received well despite the doubting Thomases who had predicted that nobody would watch and it would be a flop. However, all *of us at* Breakfast Time *were apprehensive in case* TV-am *should snatch viewers back from us with their star presenters and high-powered programme planners and editors.*

Newscaster Andrew Harvey (whom I knew well from Bristol) and I presented the French part of the programme from a high building above the city of Paris, linking up with Selina Scott and Frank Bough in the studio in London. We had flown over the afternoon before, and overnight I had used my fashion contacts – which was difficult on a Sunday – to put together and rehearse models, clothes and accessories. We started rehearsals with London at 4.30 a.m. and were on air by six.

The outside broadcast crew and I had little or no sleep, but were thrilled with the results. When put to music, the several fashion pieces were lively and colourful and must have helped keep our viewing figures up.

Sadly, back in London Selina Scott didn't seem to share our enthusiasm and by the end of the programme indicated that she found fashion confusing and something of a bore. Her indifference upset us after all our efforts back in Paris. Nowadays, as I watch her present the successful Clothes Show *programme, I think of so many fashion reporters I know who would have given their eye teeth for the job.*

My own presentation that morning didn't go unnoticed. I was delighted to be asked by the BBC to make the daily fashion reports during Ascot Week later that year.

Back in Battersea, my happy day continues with Rosemary and her baby calling to see me. Alexander is hungry, but as Rosemary undoes her blouse to put him to her breast I feel a pang of jealousy and enviously watch as she cradles him to her.

Later, Sue phones from America. She is uncomfortable in her early pregnancy, and describes the annoying symptoms of throbbing boobs and nausea. When she asks me how I am, I tell her I too have nausea and throbbing breasts! She's not sure whether she likes the idea of being pregnant – it hadn't been

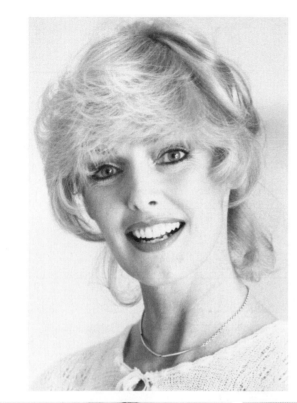

Modelling in the seventies. (Courtesy Liberty's and Brabantia.)

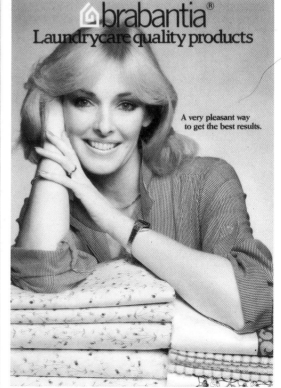

brabantia®
Laundrycare quality products

A very pleasant way
to get the best results.

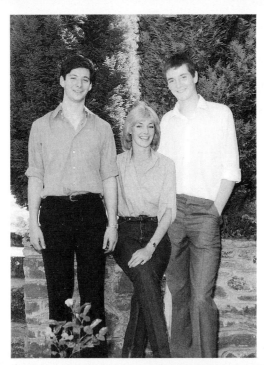

Left: Nic and Tim grown up.
Below: The Greenie Geenie in *Alladin* at the Beck Theatre, Hayes. (Courtesy Beck Theatre.)

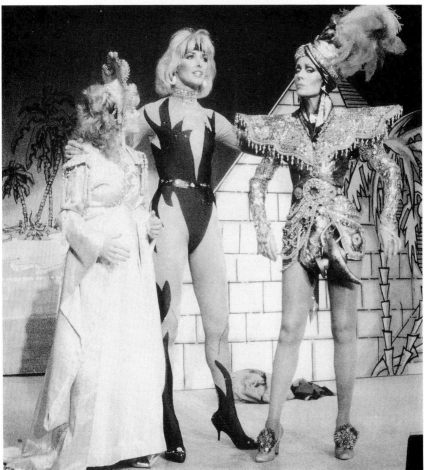

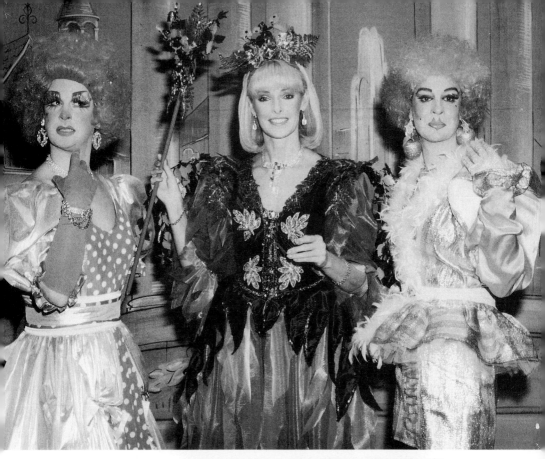

Above: The Fairy Godmother in *Cinderella* at the White Rock Theatre, Hastings. (Courtesy White Rock Theatre.)
Right: With boyfriend Peter on board the *Canberra* keeping the passengers fit.

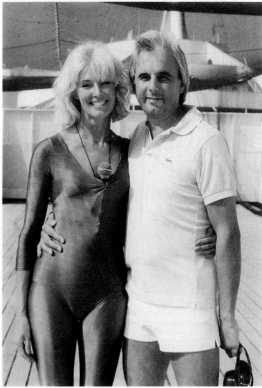

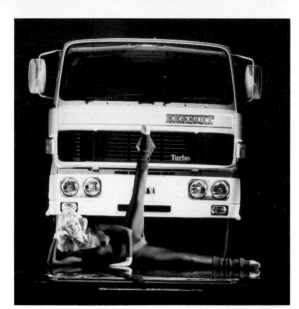

Left: Promoting Renault Trucks at the Motor Show. (Courtesy Renault Trucks.)
Below: Cover Girl in the eighties. (Courtesy Woman's Realm.)

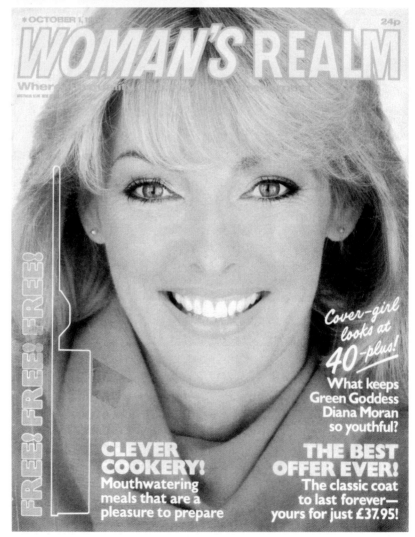

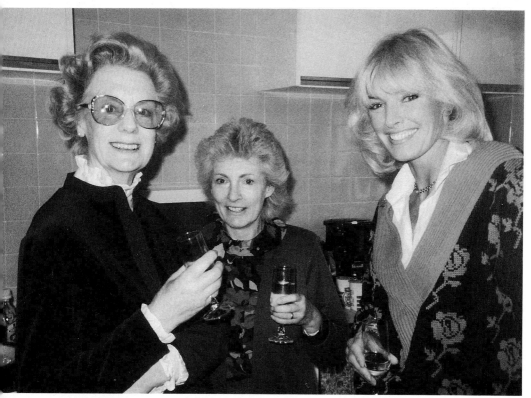

Above: With Dorothy and Cousin Pauline.
Below: Meeting the Queen Mother at the Royal Tournament. (Courtesy Royal Tournament.)

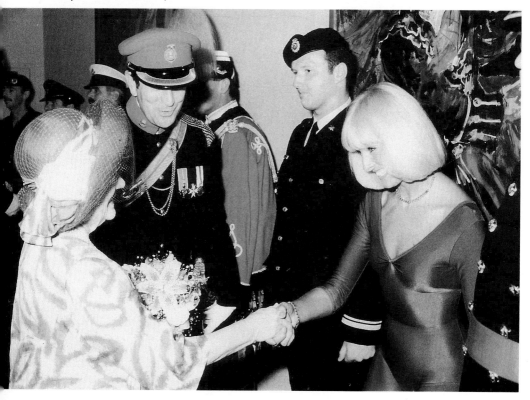

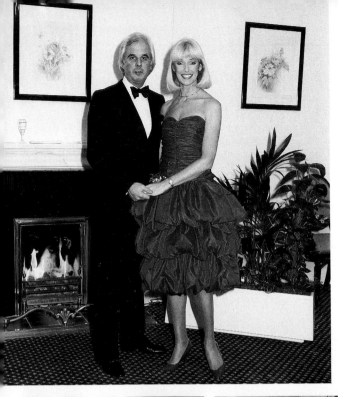

Left: With Peter, April 1988.
Below left: Maggie.
Below right: In hospital, four days after the operation.

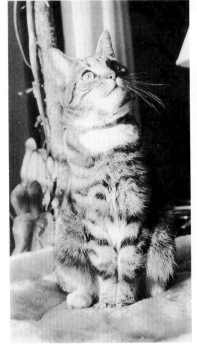

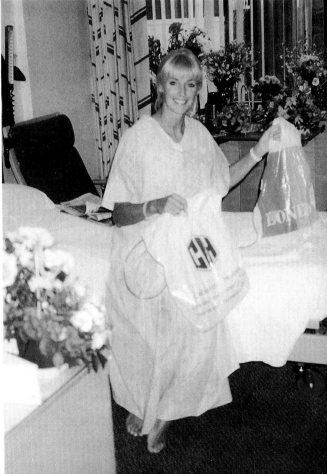

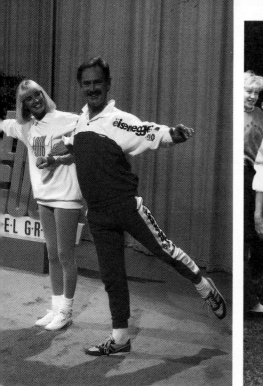
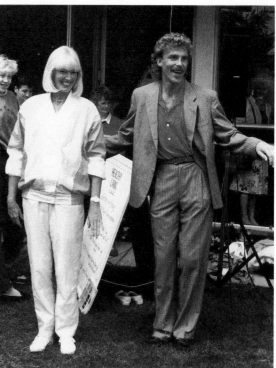

Above left: Putting Tony Adams from *Crossroads* through his paces. (Courtesy Central TV.)

Above right: My first public appearance on recovery: with 'Killer' Brian Kilcline at the Town and Country Festival at Stoneleigh. (Courtesy Central TV.)

Below left: At the opening of London Central YMCA's new training and development wing with the teachers of the Exercise to Music Training Course. (Courtesy YMCA.)

Below right: Back in Action. (Courtesy Help the Aged.)

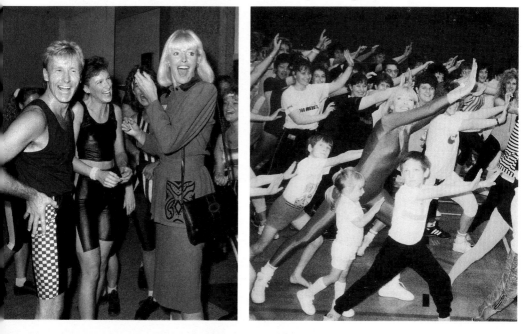

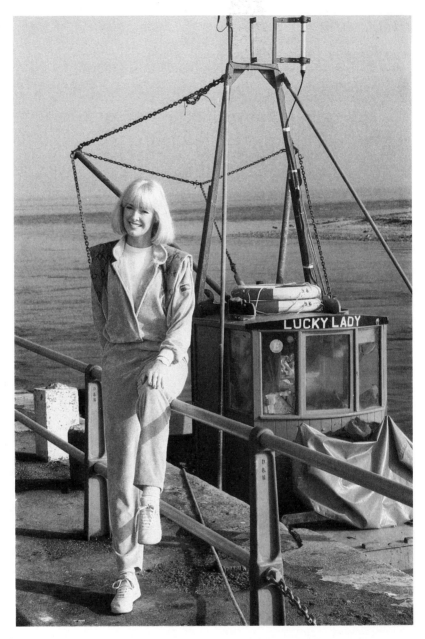

Mudeford Quay, October 1988.

in the master plan to have a baby quite so soon. She's been so successful with her horses, and she must find it frustrating to be parted from them, especially after her recent successes in racing. But I'm sure she will eventually be pleased, and cope with her new situation.

Of course, modern girls can have the choice of planning their pregnancies. I'm secretly glad I was at the tail end of the time when the old-fashioned thought was that, having kept yourself a virgin till marriage, you were God-blessed to be pregnant, and rearranged your life accordingly.

I became pregnant with Tim at twenty and loved being such a young mum, although I suppose I was only an overgrown child myself. I felt myself grow up with and through my two little boys, and found I could happily join in with their childish activities since I had only recently left mine.

Tim's birth had been quite an awakening for me, not having a mother to ask advice from and being the first of my crowd to be pregnant. I tried to find out all I could in advance. But is a woman ever really prepared for what happens to her body in childbirth? Of course, we know it's 'natural', but the theory seems very different when it has to be put into practice. And, of course, there's no going back or stopping halfway if you don't like it.

Tim decided to arrive precisely on the predicted date. John took me into hospital during the night. I was put in a small ante-room and told to sleep until the morning, when it was thought that the baby would make its appearance. But Tim was impatient, and as I walked in the darkness of my small room, trying to cope with the labour pains, I suddenly grabbed hold of the end of the bed in agony. There and then he made his dramatic appearance – much to the horror of the nurse, who heard my screams.

A day later, as I lay recovering, he was brought to my bedside by a nurse, accompanied by a specialist. They unwrapped my tightly bound bundle who, unknown to me, had been born with his feet bent upwards against his shins. He had obviously been squashed awkwardly in my womb – no wonder he'd wanted to get out in such a hurry. I was told he would not be crippled, but the whole thing took me by complete surprise and I was very upset. However, I was assured that physiotherapy and massage over the years would correct the problem, and fortunately it soon did.

What agonies we parents go through with our offspring! I recall how, at two and a half, Nic had a simple tonsil operation to help prevent his rather too numerous chest and throat infections. Sleeping in the bed next to him in hospital, I helped nurse him back to health. He soon made a speedy recovery and after a few days we returned home. He was an active, lively child, lovable but somewhat mischievous, and it was difficult to keep him still for long.

Two weeks after the operation I awoke and found him restless in his small bed. I gave him a drink of water, but to my surprise he brought back a deep red liquid. Frightened, I called the doctor, and soon an ambulance was on its way. I cradled his body in my arms as he continued to bring up blood. He had suffered a secondary haemorrhage. His little face was waxen and he was barely conscious on arrival at the hospital as they whisked him off to theatre.

The emergency over, my small blond son lay with the red transfusion tubes feeding him fresh blood. Only the day before I had given my regular pint of blood at the local church hall in Bristol. When he was strong enough to comprehend what was going on, I explained that he was receiving some of Mummy's blood, which he had often seen me giving. Since that was a normal sight, he wasn't quite so frightened. But throughout his childhood his constant nightmare was described as a mass of red snakes coming to get him.

And talking of my younger son, it's twenty-five years ago tomorrow that he was born. The summer of 1963 was beautiful, not like this awful weather. Nic, like Tim, was born during the night, though in less traumatic a fashion. I had been in labour since tea-time. As he was about to make his entrance into the world, the midwife suggested Swithin as a name since *it was 15 July, St Swithin's Day. With a final push from me he arrived, and to everyone's amusement rained water from his own little spout over the unsuspecting doctor. But all too late. It was by then five minutes past midnight, and Nicholas was to be his name.*

Saturday, 16 July

Two weeks on from the operation I look around me – the flowers are dead, but *I'm* well and truly alive. I'm still sore, but getting used to my new self. I look quite good this morning, corsetless after my bath, but I must pull my shoulders back. My posture has temporarily gone to pot, because I've a tendency to lift my shoulders up and forward – I suppose to protect myself.

Strange how my flat has become a 'home' during the last few weeks. Before, it has always been a place to rush in and out of. A place to put my head down, sleep and be off again. I realize I've 'perched' here till now, but suddenly I feel I've nested and that's good.

I'm beginning to get interested in my work and everyday life again. My post is full of newsletters from various factions of the keep-fit business. They seem to be at loggerheads with one another over teachers' training, videos, books and equipment. I sit back and feel disappointed that the hype and money-making businesses may kill off the enjoyment and subsequent benefit to the ordinary person in the street trying to keep fit. Exercising should be fun.

Two embarrassing magazine articles about the super-fit Green Goddess have been brought to my notice. I haven't given any interviews for them, or given my permission for the articles to be published; neither have I had special photographs taken. It's a bit of a nerve, really, recycling old interviews – and it irritates me to think that the public assume I make thousands from magazine and newspaper articles. I wish I did, but I won't receive a penny for these.

Sunday, 17 July

I've got to be bright today for Victoria, at seventeen the younger of my brother's two girls. I haven't seen her for three or four years.

She arrives full of beans – I've a feeling there's a bit of me in her somewhere. We have an amusing morning together, catching up on the events of the past few years. Victoria's an intelligent girl who has won a scholarship to Clifton College, the boys' public school in Bristol, where Tim and Nic went. She's in the sixth form and loving it, being one of the first girls there. She's excited at the prospect of going off to Mexico City for a month on an exchange with the school, who adopted a school there after the earthquake and tragedies of two years ago.

Victoria is fun to talk to, and I'm glad both she and her sister Lucy have decided to come and visit me. I hope we'll all keep in touch in the future. I'm sad that since my separation five years ago, and subsequent divorce – the first on either side of the family – I haven't seen or heard from most of the relations on my father's side.

Before the split, I carefully contacted all my family, and those close friends who didn't already know, to tell them of the news before the papers did. I didn't want them to be embarrassed, and once the press started – inevitably – ringing them for comments I wanted them to be prepared.

But the news, even though it was received in a hand-written letter, did come as a shock to most of the relations. I was telling them I was about to walk out on what seemed to be a perfect marriage with a kind, loving husband and two fine young adult sons. But for ten years John and I had known that the marriage was floundering – we had held it together, in the eyes of the world, until the boys were grown up and independent. Perhaps that was our mistake – putting a good face on things. Only our very closest friends knew of the breakdown of our relationship.

No one really knows what goes on within a marriage except the two partners themselves. Perhaps we should have been more open with each other about our feelings. My relations judged me by what they saw, which was not the whole truth. If you lead a conventional life, it's so easy to damn others for doing what appear to be outrageous things. And the fact that John and I remained friends may have confused the issue further. They just couldn't understand that marriage was no longer possible between us, though friendship was – and they don't seem to have forgiven me for it.

Monday, 18 July

I'm back at the Royal Marsden to have my stitches removed. A Turkish doctor has been invited to watch this time. Removing the stitches isn't as painful as I'd expected, and everyone seems pleased with the results. One of my breasts is hurting a little more than the other, and there's a lot of uncomfortable pulling going on under my arm. The surgeons tell me to massage even more to keep the skin soft and help circulation and healing. They tell me I can start doing some simple exercises and go to Mudeford to convalesce.

At home, I feel happier with the stitches out and tackle simple tasks around the flat with renewed vigour. Cautiously, I begin to exercise.

My favourite form of exercise, when I have time, is to join a class taken by Lucy Jackson, who teaches the Medau method of whole body movement. It contrasts with and complements the static exercises that, due to restricted space, I usually perform on stage or in a television studio. The Medau method has me running, leaping and dancing across a room, using up space. I find it therapeutic and it helps release my inhibitions and emotions.

Lucy calls to see me this afternoon with Lala, her daughter. They both know I've been unwell and I decide to confide in them. Lucy is blonde and vibrant, in her fifties and a shining example of a life-long keep-fitter. Lala has benefited from her mother's enthusiasm, and I know from seeing her in class that she has a beautiful, supple and efficient body. She looks blooming – her first baby is due next week.

I wish I'd known all I do now when I was expecting my babies. There's so much that women can do to help themselves to recover more quickly. By watching one's diet and taking the correct exercise before and immediately after pregnancy, many gynaecological problems can be avoided for the future. It's so simple today to ask for advice or to read the masses of literature available to help oneself and one's family enjoy better health. I found out the hard way . . .

When I exercise, it has four or five immediate benefits on my body. They all begin with S.

The first is suppleness. *It's something we all need to work at, especially as we get older. It's good to be able to use our bodies efficiently, extending them fully, bending, stretching and reaching. By maintaining maximum mobility for as many years as possible we help retain our physical independence into very old age.*

Through exercise, we build up stamina: *stamina to sustain full, free bodily movement for as long as we require it, without feeling puffed, exhausted or faint. Correct exercising should help our circulation and strengthen and improve the lung and heart functions.*

Regular exercising makes us stronger. *It builds up our muscles, including those of the heart, enabling the heart and lungs to give added performance. It's particularly important for sportspeople, to enable them to reach their peak.*

We learn skill *through exercise. In other words, whatever we attempt to do, we do it with control, co-ordinating mind and body.*

And the fifth S stands for sex. *Through exercise, and with all the other benefits I've mentioned, one's sex life can be enjoyed more fully.*

I'm often asked what are the best forms of exercise and how much and how often we should do it. A good basic rule is twenty minutes, three times a week. That can be simply twenty minutes' brisk walk, enough to make us feel a little bit puffed.

The average person wants a little of all the S's I've just mentioned, but we must work out for ourselves our individual aims and requirements. We're all made differently – large, tall, short, fat – and we can't alter our basic frame. Being slim, too, doesn't necessarily mean being fit. Having said that, however, many people in Britain are overweight, and an increase in years should not necessarily mean an increase in the waistline.

One of the best ways to get motivated is to get the eating pattern right. Healthy eating and exercise go hand in hand – you can't have one without the other. By shedding a little extra weight, more mobility can be achieved and progress made. But choosing what food to eat and what exercise to take must be a serious decision – one that becomes a pleasurable pattern for life, and not just a five-minute wonder.

So much has been written about a sensible diet that I almost hesitate to add more. Most people already know the obvious things – lots of fibre, nuts and pulses, and fresh fruit and vegetables; less red meat, fat, sugar, starch and salt. Grill food where possible, rather than frying or roasting, and trim off excess fat first. When you do need to use fat or oil, make sure it's a polyunsaturated vegetable oil and not animal fat. Drink, by all means, but sparingly – alcohol is bursting with calories. Dry white wine is a good friend because it's relatively low in calories and doesn't make you seem like a spoilsport at parties. Spirits are best left alone.

And talking of parties, we all have binges now and then. But be intelligent about it, and next day drink lots of water but don't eat much. Have an all-fruit day occasionally (I do). And if you suspect that your careful, health-conscious, weight-aware diet might be lacking anything, take multi-vitamin pills on a regular basis or have a check-up with your doctor. It's especially important for vegetarians, who can easily miss out on certain vitamins and minerals.

I'm a stickler for breakfast – it's essential. Whether my

day starts at 10 a.m. or 4 a.m., I always make myself a light, healthy meal that will give me a constant energy level. Even if I don't get any lunch (which often happens on some of my more hectic days) I can last out until mid-afternoon without resorting to those fattening snacks that make for peaks and troughs of energy.

I start with fresh fruit juice (that's my vitamin C). Then I have a bowl of home-mixed low-sugar muesli (energy and fibre) with skimmed milk. A piece of wholemeal bread (more fibre) and marmalade follow. I'll eat a piece of fruit (more vitamins), and I'll drink a cup of decaffeinated coffee – again with skimmed milk, and without sugar. My one weakness is the butter I have with the bread and marmalade – well, I am a West Country girl, and I compensate by saying no to cream and chocolate!

I don't really like red meat, and I don't buy it to cook. Of course, if I'm out being entertained I'll eat what has kindly been prepared – it would be churlish to do otherwise. But Peter and I eat fish or poultry for preference. That's one of the many pleasures of having a house by the sea in Dorset – there's so much lovely fish we're spoilt for choice.

The other half of the healthy living equation is exercise, and, like dieting, it can be as pleasurable or as hard as you make it. Exercising in a class or with a partner is good fun, and you stretch more with a little help from a friend. The discipline and encouragement are good, too. I like it when people make friends in class, and notice that as they become more confident with themselves they grow more extrovert. In a good class, complexions glow and everyone seems to smile, breathe and talk in a more relaxed manner.

I feel, through sport, that barriers and prejudices can be destroyed. People who are fit and join sports clubs to make regular tennis, football, water sports or whatever part of their life seem to make more friends and share experiences as they progress and get more fit. Their social life is better and lived to the full.

It's never too soon or too late to start exercising. But I cannot stress too strongly that we're all different, and that you should *not aim too high or you will be disappointed. I've seen people injured, mentally as well as physically, through starting sport or a tough exercise class before they were fit enough. In order to keep fit, one must get fit in the first place. I always tell people to ask the experts for advice, and to shop around a little until they find a class, exercise or sport they're comfortable with. People should get to know their limitations and shouldn't use equipment without supervision. The important rule is always to warm up at the beginning of a session, gradually build up the amount of exercise, and then cool down at the end of it. It's common sense, really. People shouldn't take themselves too seriously, either, unless of course they're involved in competitive sports. Exercise should be fun.*

Over the past twenty years I have conscientiously looked after my health. I'm aware I can't add years to my life, but by discovering and treating my cancer at this early stage I hope I will be adding life to my years.

Peter seems very tired again this evening – he's got so much to contend with. I ask him if he's happy, and he assures me he is. I wonder when I'll be fit enough for us to be able to get together comfortably to make love again. There are so many uncertainties. Will the bodily contact hurt me? Will my reduced femininity put Peter off? And will my lack of confidence and feelings of tension mean that I can't relax into lovemaking – which in turn will prevent Peter from relaxing and enjoying this shared experience?

Tuesday, 19 July

A better night's sleep. Each time I woke up during the night I turned over on to my other side, but was able to drop off to sleep again. I was wary but it felt reasonably comfortable, although I do feel a bit tender this morning.

I'm getting bored, and begin to think about work and the future. Perhaps I should cut my hair, have a new image and make a fresh start. The trouble is, I've already recorded pieces to go into the programme *Look Good, Feel Great.* If, when the series starts, I have a new hairstyle the pieces won't match up.

So much for peace and quiet. Maggie has decided to break my boredom and has been very sick all over the floor and bed. I'll have to change the sheets. I obviously haven't been brushing her enough, and she's sicked up a fur ball caused by all her licking and cleaning. It's a real effort to clear it up, and soon I run out of energy and climb back into bed for an afternoon nap. But the children in the flats have broken up from school and are playing noisily outside my window; I can't sleep. I feel low and depressed, and am pleased when Peter arrives home.

By nine o'clock he packs me off to bed. He tucks me up tightly but as soon as he leaves the room I burst into tears and cry myself to sleep. I feel a failure.

Wednesday, 20 July

I still feel depressed this morning and need consolation, so I creep into Peter's bed for another good cry and a cuddle.

When I have my bath, I'm upset to see the scar on my left breast is weeping and looking very red and ugly. It worries me, and I wonder if I should cancel going down to Mudeford at the weekend. What if I need the surgeons' attention? Peter doesn't help by commenting that it's sad to see me like this now, considering how well I was before the operation. I know what he means, but it's little or no consolation and makes me feel weepy again.

I grow more unhappy as the morning goes on and telephone Mr Crosswell, who asks me to come over straightaway. I tell Peter, who comes back from the office and takes me to the hospital.

I have an infection. Apparently the skin where my nipple was is very thin and has pulled apart. Mr Crosswell tells me it's very important that infections are cleared up immediately. After it's dealt with and I'm restitched I feel considerably relieved.

Thursday, 21 July

It's a black day today, the worst since the op. Everything hurts. I'm worried about the septic scar and I think the antibiotics are adding to my depression. Tearfully, I go back to bed for the afternoon but I can't sleep.

I'm woken by a man delivering some beautiful flowers from Annie and her angels. My mood lifts, and I'm delighted when Rosemary and her baby call to see me again. Rosemary's upset, as she can see I've been crying and knows it's not like me. But over a cup of tea the blues disappear.

Peter comes home and decides to surprise me by taking me out to an Italian restaurant. What a nice treat. But within an hour my breasts begin to feel uncomfortable and I know it's time for bed. I have enjoyed my outing, however, and sense I'm on the road to recovery.

Friday, 22 July

A better night's sleep. My spirits are high and I'm thinking positive. I've had enough of slopping around in a tracksuit – I'll dress up and look smart to visit Mr Crosswell this morning. I put on a navy and white outfit and give myself a lift with a pair of high heels.

He's pleased the infection is subsiding, but says it would be better for me not to go to Mudeford this weekend. I'm sad for Peter, who's been looking forward to getting a break. But personally I'm relieved because I know the journey would have caused me considerable discomfort.

Saturday, 23 July

I'm tired of sleeping on my own and, waking early, crawl into Peter's bed. We cautiously make love like two prickly hedge-hogs. I'm overjoyed to find that my fears for this moment are unfounded. All the familiar closeness and tenderness are still there, and so is the passion – though it's a different kind of passion, with even greater warmth than before. I find I'm crying, but this time, for once, they are tears of joy.

As the day wears on, however, I begin to get depressed and frustrated by all the things I'm still not able to do. Peter tries his hardest to keep my spirits up, but as we watch the Royal Tournament on television I think back to the fun I had last year as the Blue Goddess. How super-fit I'd felt and what a success it had all been, as in front of an audience of seventeen thousand the Navy and I jumped into action. I'm amused to see and hear my same choice of music, 'Jump', used for this year's audience participation spot, and take it as a compliment.

Sunday, 24 July

A sunny day, and I wake up determined to be better. We make love, with a little more confidence than yesterday.

Peter decides to take me out to another Italian restaurant in the Fulham Road for lunch. We go at 12.30 to avoid the crush, and I feel fine. But after an hour and a half the pain returns to my chest, my skin begins to tighten and I know it's time to go.

Peter calls for the bill just as a group of young people come in and sit down at the next table. One of the girls is Koo Stark, with whom we'd spent a week doing a promotion in Crete last year. I say hello to her but feel jealous of her youth, her looks and her future. Just for a minute I feel mine is slipping away and that I'm ageing fast. But I pull back my shoulders, get up elegantly from the table and walk tall to the door, hoping Koo won't suspect anything's wrong. How fortunate it is we're not able to see into the future.

When we return, friends from Mudeford have left a message on my answerphone. People are beginning to ask where we are.

Monday, 25 July

Dressed in my smart scarlet suit I cheerfully take a taxi, alone, to the hospital. Each time I go I hope I'm not recognized so that my secret can remain a secret.

Mr Scott and Mr Crosswell check that everything is OK, but instead of removing the stitches, as I'd expected, put in another three. This means I'll have to stay in London a little longer.

Back in the flat I ring Lucy for news of Lala's baby, but it hasn't arrived yet.

Tuesday, 26 July

Both boys continue to telephone regularly to find out how I am. They'll never quite know how important their calls are.

My breasts are very painful today and appear a bit crumpled. I massage in some calendula cream, hoping it will work miracles but fearing it may not. It worries me, not that I've been mutilated, but that my reincarnation could be crumbling and my dreams disintegrating, which would seem unfair – a bit like being given a taste of honey and then having it taken away. Mr Scott said he used to recommend Oil of Ulay to soften the skin. It made him laugh when I told him I was the Oil of Ulay lady in the television ads a few years ago.

I've been catching up with all the viewing I've been wanting to do over the past few years but have been too busy to do. Now, though, I'm getting square eyes watching so much television and so many videos. Perhaps I should write a book. Friends have been telling me for years to write about my varied life. On Peter's suggestion, I've kept this detailed diary from the day I was told my bad news. He felt it would be therapeutic for me. Maybe this will be my starting point.

Wednesday, 27 July

A much better night. I've finished the antibiotics, so I feel more chirpy.

Offers of work are coming in, but Annie fends off enquiries about jobs before September. I'm offered a public work-out for October, but decline. I'm sure I can't get physically fit by then – not enough to motivate and lead several hundred people, and to be watched and criticized. However, I do have a date in November, and I will be fit enough for that. It's my goal to aim for. I giggle at the thought of the many clients who have been told I'm unavailable or away. They must think I'm having a wonderful long holiday this year. If only they knew – and if only I was.

Elizabeth arrives to take me to Mr Crosswell. I discuss the crumpling with him as he removes some of my stitches, but he tells me to be patient, to get on with my life and let time be the healer. He advises me to direct my interest away from myself, which is easier said than done. With the constant gnawing pain and my restricted movement I'm like a caged animal waiting to break out. I'm only too aware there's a whole lot of living to be done, and Peter deserves a bit of pampering himself. I want to be independent. I hate being beholden to others.

Mr Crosswell tells me to go away and enjoy myself and do all the things I want to do. I resolve to do as I'm told. When he's taken the last stitches out, in a few days' time, I won't have to see a doctor again – unless it's absolutely necessary, of course – until late September.

As I leave his surgery, I remember my posture. I pull back my shoulders and stand up tall. It hurts my chest. Nevertheless, I'm going to keep standing up straight and enjoy the rest of the summer and the fresh air in Mudeford.

So far I've managed to keep all this from the press. I'm so pleased that my trusted friends and family haven't squeaked and let my secret out. At the time of my divorce, too, they joined ranks and protected me.

I've given hundreds of interviews to the press over the past few years, most of them free. The BBC would tell me which interviews they wished me to do, and more recently Central TV have done the same for the new programme. I recall the first time I was interviewed by Jean Rook in the *Daily Express*.

On that occasion she had been kind to me (later on, over my divorce, she was not). She had asked me if there was anything about myself I'd like to change. My boobs, I replied. How ironical. She then asked me how I would feel as I got older and lost my shape, but I commented that, with correct diet and exercise, my figure shouldn't change and increase with the years. But I hadn't bargained for something like this, and I'm determined to get myself back into shape as soon as possible. Only then, looking good and feeling great, will I be prepared to tell the press my story. Maybe it could be of help and encouragement to the many other women who will be told they have breast cancer.

Thursday, 28 July

I'm still sleeping in the spare room on the sofa bed. This room, with its glorious view over the Thames, is usually my dining room. But it's great as a bedroom, and when I wake up in the night I can sit and watch the reflected lights of London twinkling in the water outside my window.

The river has a life of its own, and early in the morning the cormorants and herons join the many ducks in their search for fish and other tit-bits. A flock of Canada geese gather noisily under my window, and the swans float effortlessly in and out of the colourful houseboats moored opposite. It's amazingly peaceful my side of the river, though throughout the night the constant distant buzz of traffic can be heard along the Embankment on the north side. At high tide the chug-chug-chug of small tugs can be heard as they miraculously pull behind them two huge barges loaded down with container after container, thirty or more, full of London's rubbish, which they take away downstream.

My agent asks me to telephone an American fitness expert, who would like to meet me whilst he's here in London. He sounds nice and we chatter on, comparing the health and fitness business in America and England. I promise we'll meet on his next visit over here. Little does he realize the state I'm in just now, and I'm sure he'd be very surprised if he knew the truth. However, his call boosts my morale and makes me appreciate I haven't lost everything. I still have my reputation.

Peter rings at five o'clock to enquire if I'm all right. He's on what I laughingly call a boys' day out – a group of invited businessmen together on a social event. I expect him home at seven, but the hire car delivers him back at nine, a bit 'tired and emotional'. I pretend to be cross but soften when he tells me he loves me a lot, that we're in this mess together, and that together we'll pull through.

Friday, 29 July

Peter tells me he has spoken – confidentially, of course – to a well-known and respected figure in the publishing world, Harold Evans, and has arranged to see him next week. I decide I definitely will try writing a book. At last I've a project to work on, something to keep my brain occupied and to break the monotony.

Gleefully, I spend the morning preparing for Mudeford. I shall be pleased to have a change of scenery – I'm very attached to the flat, but I've seen rather a lot of it recently. Luckily for me, the weather in the last few weeks has been a record of awfulness, so I haven't missed much and have stayed cool. Hot weather would have made my discomfort much worse.

I pack the minimum of clothes – just tracksuits – the contents of the fridge and, of course, the cat. Peter puts it all in the car and arranges me in the back, with pillows all around for support. Even so, I still feel most of the bumps and turns of the road, and by Lyndhurst, in the New Forest, I've had enough. It's been a long, uncomfortable three hours, not helped by Maggie crying in her box most of the time. Unusually, we've both disliked this journey.

But it's good to arrive. The sea air smells invigorating, the house is in order and the garden looks colourful too. Peter's mother has put some flowers in a vase, which makes it instantly feel like home. Tentatively, Peter enquires if I could manage a trip to the local Indian restaurant for an early supper.

I wasn't prepared for this and feel nervous, but I'm determined to clock up a first. We stop to chat to lots of local people, and afterwards, coming out of the restaurant, decide to go for an evening walk along the quay. I'm thrilled to be doing normal things again.

Bed-time comes early and we sleep together in the same room for the first time since the operation. I begin to realize there *is* life after cancer, and sleep very soundly.

Saturday, 30 July

After a loving start, we coast through an easy day with Peter's mother keeping me company whilst he shops. Roy, a neighbour, calls with a salmon caught yesterday. Several other friends, seeing us sitting by the window, drop in to say hello. The local people are so friendly – that's the beauty of Mudeford. Supper – Roy's fresh salmon and garden vegetables – tastes wonderful.

I spend a quiet afternoon relaxing and listening to music. Sounds bring back such strong memories. Hearing Widor's organ toccata, I recall attending the boys' concert in the school hall when Tim was about eleven.

He had been taking recorder and piano lessons and getting on quite well, so I was hoping to see him perform along with the other pupils. A young lad finished playing the violin and the music master introduced the next boy, whom he told us we wouldn't see but only hear, since the organ console was at the back of the hall. To my amazement, the beautiful sounds of the toccata were played competently by Tim, who, having been attracted to the powerful sound of the organ, had secretly pestered the organist to give him private tuition. The organist had made special blocks to help Tim's little legs reach the pedals. John and I were full of pride.

His enthusiasm continued until university, when his studies, coupled with his naval commitments, took priority. Two years ago, whilst serving on a small submarine, his musical interest was reawakened by the sound of the Royal Marine Band and he decided to learn another, more mobile, pipe instrument. At his suggestion, his Christmas present from me that year was a set of bagpipes. I never did learn what his fellow sailors thought of his practising in the confines of a submarine. I really must ask him some time.

Sunday, 31 July

Today I feel close to Peter and very loved. In the bright summer sunshine, we walk hand in hand to our local, the Haven, for a glass of wine and a crab sandwich. It's good to see the harbour and quayside full of holidaymakers. We sit outside the pub and watch the world go by, talking to many of the locals. It feels pleasant to get involved again, and as I pick up the threads of life my worries seem far behind me.

AUGUST

Monday, 1 August

It's 5 a.m. and we're on our way back to London. What a shame. Lying down on the back seat seems to be a more comfortable position to travel in, and enables me to catch up on some lost sleep.

Back in the flat I unpack, then breakfast and bath. But by one o'clock I'm exhausted and flop into bed. I'm amazed to find it's five o'clock when I wake up again, as Annie calls with more details of work coming in for me. She gives me the schedule of recordings for *Look Good, Feel Great*, which I'll be presenting for Central TV in Birmingham. I'm to start on 8 September in the studio. Even though there's no jumping up and down involved, I feel a little uneasy and apprehensive. I've just got to be right by then.

I decide it's time to take back the responsibility for domesticity and I make supper. At bed-time, I return to the double bed and Peter. Pleasant as it was, I've had enough of being on my own in the spare room.

Tuesday, 2 August

It's over a month since the operation, and finally the last of the stitches is removed. A message on my answerphone has told me Lala's baby has arrived. It's a girl, named Harriet. So from Mr Crosswell's consulting rooms off Oxford Street I walk to the Portland Hospital to deliver a present for her.

The place is jumping with photographers in the street outside, hoping to catch a glimpse of Fergie, due to arrive here any day for the birth of her baby. I stride confidently in and out of the hospital and am recognized by several of the photographers.

I hail a taxi to take me to Ian, my hairdresser. He's kind and understanding, but soon I begin to ache from all the effort, the taxi journey and sitting in one position in his salon. However, Peter collects me as we've arranged and I'm thankful to get home. I lie on the floor, which seems to give me some relief from the gnawing pains around my chest and under my arms. I've been trying to do without sleeping pills or painkillers for a week or so, but it's no good tonight – I need both. So as not to disturb Peter, I trundle myself back into the spare bedroom and have a very poor night's sleep.

Wednesday, 3 August

I still ache from my activity of the last few days, but decide it's time I washed my own hair. The washing proves quite easy, but the blow drying is more uncomfortable and exhausting. At least I've done it myself.

Dressed in my Florida tracksuit, with my hair squeaky clean, I feel more confident when my new publisher arrives to see me, as arranged. We discuss a possible book.

I speak to the boys on the phone, and they both sound in good form. Tim is off soon on a trip to America, taking naval cadets first to Washington and then to a naval base in Canada. Nic tells me he's looking for a flat of his own and seems busy in his work. I tell them both about the book to sound them out, indicating they'll feature in it. They say it seems like a good idea, and they know it will keep me busy and therefore happy.

Later, as I talk to Lucy about Lala and her new granddaughter, she too agrees I ought to write a book about the past few months of my life. Married to a gynaecologist, she tells me she has many friends and acquaintances who, in their fifties and sixties, have had breast cancer. She feels many women could be helped by a book written by someone who has gone through the experience herself.

I'm upset to learn from my agent that the scheduling of the transmission of the second series of *Look Good, Feel Great* is uncertain. Coverage of the Olympic Games has changed everything. We have already filmed lots of interesting items which are planned to be inserted into the programmes.

The first series, shown last year, was important to me. I decided to make a conscious effort to re-establish myself as Diana Moran, television presenter, and not just be the Green Goddess. I didn't want my identity completely dominated by the green lady, and to be committed to jumping up and down for the rest of my career. I knew I was taking a risk by not appearing in green, but it seemed to work. I do hope the powers that be get the schedules sorted out soon. The programme was so well received by the public.

Thursday, 4 August

The Queen Mother's birthday, and my own mother's birthday. I never forget.

I'm feeling good today and very positive. I decide to do the ironing and find there's lots of it. I cook myself some lunch and settle down to a video, but I'm very happy to be interrupted when Rosemary pops in for a short time to see me with young Alexander, who's growing fast. She's been a wonderful support.

Liz Calder, my publisher, calls and we confirm that I will go ahead with the book. However, copy is needed by October, so I'll have to work fast – but then I love a challenge, and I have time on my hands. Now I must find a typist.

Philip, my accountant, telephones. He too, I learn, has been in hospital. After two months he has returned to work, and realizes from looking at my erratic accounts that all is not well with me. I explain the position and he tells me I will need to be very frugal in the coming months.

My breasts feel more comfortable today than they have done

for the last month. The scars on the one side are nearly healed, and I look almost normal. The other side, though, is still badly bruised.

Friday, 5 August

I've so much to do today as I get everything ready to go down to Mudeford for a month or so's recuperation. My fairy godmother, Elizabeth, calls to say goodbye to me. I open one of my half-bottles of champagne to celebrate my speedy recovery, much of which is due to her help and encouragement.

The weather is fine and my journey more comfortable. Sitting upright with the seat belt tight across my chest doesn't appeal to me, so once again I lie in the back of the car.

On our arrival we walk around the quay and, passing the local fish stall, stop to talk to our fishmonger friend John Batchelor. We return home with lobsters, which I prepare for supper.

Saturday, 6 August

The local florist arrives with a colourful arrangement which Philip has sent to make me feel at home. Peter does the weekend shopping while I take it quietly. I potter around the house doing odd jobs, but can't quite get up enough strength to attend to the garden. After a snack lunch we relax outside, but it's too hot for me to sit out with my corset and tracksuit on.

Later, as we get ready for an evening out with friends, I feel nervous. My dress, the only one which covers up my corset, looks dowdy and ill-fitting. I've forgotten to bring my summer shoes, and I fiddle with my jewellery. I feel very insecure, but Peter reassures me and tells me I don't look the freak I feel.

Apprehensively I follow him into the bar of the local hotel where we have arranged to meet. It's full of people and noise, but everyone is nice and enquires where we have been. I soon relax amongst friends, and later we head off to the Chinese restaurant, where a big table has been booked for us all to celebrate a friend's fortieth birthday.

Peter drops me off at the door, where I'm welcomed by Doreen, who works behind the bar. She has two of Maggie's beautiful offspring for her pets and I enquire after them.

Supper is fun, but by the end of the first course I begin to feel tired and the gnawing pain returns to my chest. I decide I need to go home, so politely excuse myself. I can't sustain my energy for too long yet.

Sunday, 7 August

I decide I simply must tackle the garden. I dead-head the pansies and the antirrhinums, and looking at the poor performance of the roses, covered in black spot, decide they will have to come out soon. But I don't feel strong enough to do that today. All too soon I begin to grow tired, so I sit down to weed and prune. I finish by giving the garden a good watering with the hose. But I feel so frustrated – there's so much more to be done.

I ask Peter to help me clear up, after which we decide to go for a walk. The exercise improves my circulation and makes me forget my aches and pains. We walk along Avon Beach and watch the holidaymakers enjoying themselves. The weather is beautiful and people are busy windsurfing, water-skiing, boating and fishing. We return along the beach to the quay, where we stop to buy some crab for tonight's supper.

Monday, 8 August

I sleep through till four o'clock, and then clock-watch till Peter is woken by his alarm at five. He leaves at 5.30 to catch the fast train from Christchurch to Waterloo. By going so early he hopes to be in the office by his usual eight o'clock. Poor man, I hope he can sleep a bit on the train. Not that I envy his fellow passengers, with his awful snoring.

I look out at a beautiful morning and see the fishermen going about their business. And even a few holidaymakers are up taking a six o'clock stroll around the quay.

So here I am, alone at last in Mudeford to convalesce and regain my strength. The day is beautiful – the English summer has finally arrived. We haven't had it so hot since June, when I was doing all that travelling to the West Country by car. What a lot has happened to me since then . . .

After tidying the house, I do the washing in my splendid new machine. Next I fill up the large watering can and try to water my window boxes and tubs. But it's a mistake. The can is too heavy for me to manoeuvre, and it hurts. I won't do that again in a hurry. I move on to fork loosely over the top soil in the front garden, but I find that a bit 'iffy' too. Peter's mother calls to make certain I'm all right. Douglas, my charming next-door neighbour, offers to do my heavy shopping, and Rhonda kindly phones with details of local typists and word processor operators, which I had asked her about on Saturday night. Several of my other friends telephone to make sure I've settled in well and have all I need.

Because the sunshine's too good to miss I decide to redesign one of my corsets to allow me to wear some cooler clothing. On the oldest one, I mark a line with pencil and cut it down to shape. As I do, I'm reminded of my mother and all the sewing she did – it's one thing she taught me to do really well. Why do some people take their mothers so much for granted? Young people all too easily dismiss their elders by thinking they're too old and out of touch. But age means experience, and mothers mean security.

I fetch my sewing machine from the cupboard, but find it's difficult to carry and get irritated that everything takes me twice as long as usual. I sit at the machine and put the finishing touches to my redesigned corset. I must get the surgeons to recommend the design to the manufacturers. I slip the finished article on and decide it looks good and that the necessary support is still there. I often secretly thought I'd like to be a dress designer.

Joan, another of my kind neighbours, calls with some wide elastic she has found from which I can make a boob tube, to wear under my swimsuit and tops for short periods. I'll need it if the weather gets any hotter.

Arriving back in the early evening, Peter is dismayed to find me exhausted. I've done too much too soon. He's brought with him from London the *Evening Standard*, which I settle down and read. The television and papers are full of Fergie's baby, Beatrice, born at 8.18 today, the 8th of the 8th '88. A lucky omen.

Tim had been a midshipman at Dartmouth at the same time as Prince Andrew, and both had continued their training on HMS *Intrepid* and HMS *Invincible*. At the midshipmen's passing out parade and on open days at sea the Queen and Prince Philip attended in the same way as we other parents did, all mingling together and watching, with interest and pride, the progress of our respective sons.

Tuesday, 9 August

Peter leaves at the crack of dawn, but I slumber on till eight o'clock. I take my breakfast into the garden and enjoy it in the morning sunshine. Then I construct an ad for an audio typist.

Telephoning the local newspaper, the *Bournemouth Echo*, I'm amused by the girl taking the details. She thinks she may like the job herself. She's leaving to get married, so checks with her fiancé, but he decides she will be taking on too much, what with the honeymoon, decorating their new home etc. Shame – she sounds so nice. She tells me my ad will appear on Thursday and Friday this week.

It seems everyone is checking up on me today. Peter's mother calls with the stamps I wanted and some fresh beans. Neville and Peg, more local friends, bring me home-grown tomatoes, a cucumber and some red peppers. Roy calls in with another fish, a fresh lettuce and a huge marrow. The joys of country living! I write some letters and take myself for a short walk to the postbox, but I feel hot and uncomfortable and can't get used to this weather. Judy phones from Bristol, Elizabeth from London, and Derek's wife, Audrey, rings to ask if I'd like to go and stay in Somerset with them for part of my convalescence.

I settle down in the shade to make my boob tube, but find my patience isn't good and again I'm frustrated. But I've lots to do – cooking, washing and sewing. With Peter staying in London, my time's my own and I use it to the full.

By bed-time I'm exhausted. I've hardly sat still all day, and I promise not to do so much tomorrow. My body is beginning to feel more comfortable, but the trouble is my energy level is low. I look at myself, tired and out of tune, and wonder where my waistline, flat tummy and tidy thighs have gone. I'm flabby and know I must soon start shaping up again in earnest.

As I lie in bed, I remember I haven't locked the French windows downstairs. Wearily, I get out of bed and try to make the house secure. But I'm overtired and I don't have the strength to push the stiff door back to lock it. After several attempts I panic, and begin to cry with frustration and rage. Damn it. But there's nothing I can do except go to bed and hope the bogey man won't come round tonight.

Wednesday, 10 August

I'm awake at 3.30, feeling uneasy because of the unlocked door. I thrash about uncomfortably and decide it's time to turn over and test sleeping on my tummy. Very gingerly, I position myself with a pillow under my chest for support. But I don't stay there long, and soon realize I'm not feeling good today. I've overdone it in the last few days and my body aches.

A sitting-down day is required. I decide to find out more about breast cancer and how to help one's recovery. I wonder if I can get details of specific exercises to regain my mobility. Looking through the telephone directory at the many cancer organizations, I decide to call BACUP – the British Association of Cancer United Patients.

BACUP are particularly helpful. Breast cancer has been with us since the days of the Bible. They tell me that in England and Wales alone there are twenty-five thousand women each year with this form of the disease, and of those, fifteen thousand will die from it. It appears breast cancer is not on the increase, as many of us might think, but is more evident nowadays because modern women live longer. There are more women alive today beyond the age of fifty, when breast cancer is more likely. Years ago many of these women would have died from other, now preventable, illnesses.

As to the cause of breast cancer, it is thought the influence of hormones, in particular oestrogen, is very strong. Girls who start menstruating early, and those women who have a late menopause, show more of a tendency to develop it.

But of course nowadays breast cancer is curable, and the success rate is greater because the disease can be caught sooner, if diagnosed in time. Often no lump can be felt, as in my case. Of course, self-examination of the breasts is most important for all women. If a lump, however small, is found it should be reported to the doctor. More often than not the lump turns out to be something harmless, such as a cyst, which can be dealt with quite simply and then ignored. Often this puts an end to the scare. However, the doctor may refer his patient to a specialist who will then, after various tests, be able to give his considered opinion as to the treatment required.

In April 1988 the Government brought out a scheme to screen all women of fifty to sixty-four. A mammogram, such as I had at the clinic, shows up even the smallest of cancers – those which we ourselves and the doctors can't even feel. And this is where the success rate lies. Non-invasive breast cancers can be removed. Invasive breast cancer can be treated with greater and more positive effect, and before the cells can escape to form other possible trouble spots around the body. The plan is for each woman to be screened regularly every three years, in a similar way to screening for cervical cancer. Hopefully, the new scheme will have the same degree of success.

But, as with many things in life, we must help ourselves. Our body belongs to us alone and we must be in control of it. Even when cancer has been diagnosed there are some women who reject the advice of doctors.

I'm interested to hear a comment on *Points of View* from a woman saying she would like to hear some good news about cancer patients, not always sad. She's referring to a recent programme I decided not to watch, an excellent drama about two women dying from cancer. I was afraid that viewing it alone would depress me . . .

Peter breezes in late from his London office. He's been caught up in business. David and Rhonda ask us to join them at the Italian restaurant for a quick bite. We have common interests and get on well. They know I've been ill, but don't know it was cancer and therefore we don't have to talk about it. I feel a bit rough tonight and find I don't last the course for long, so all too soon it's home to bed for me. I sob my heart out in Peter's arms.

Thursday, 11 August

I'm puffy-eyed from crying and lack of sleep, but I must get on. Ken, my Man Friday – or should I call him my Man Thursday? – will be arriving soon to help me around the house. He's a tall, handsome West Country man, retired and in his sixties, cheery and very adaptable. He mends a plug, does the cleaning and takes me shopping for a whirly-gig clothes line – having first borrowed Douglas's from next door to see if it fits into the hole already in the garden path.

I hang out the washing cautiously, as I find it a bit of a strain on my upper arms and chest. I find the doors, cupboards and curtains need more effort to open down here in Mudeford than in my modern, touch-button London flat. The stairs here use up a lot of my energy, and I haven't yet adjusted from the ease of the flat. I soon get impatient and feel extremely tired.

I'm doing more exercise, which can't be bad, but I'm paying for being so energetic on Monday and Tuesday. Over my years involved in keep-fit I have learnt that pain from over-exertion is felt not one but two days later. Everything seems to be pulling around my chest and under my arms, and I promise myself a sit-down this afternoon.

But my quiet afternoon turns out to be amazingly busy. The advertisement in the *Bournemouth Echo* brings in dozens of telephone calls, starting just after lunch. There are obviously a lot of part-time typists in this area looking for work. It keeps my depression at bay, and I arrange to see several typists tomorrow.

I've been keeping this diary faithfully every day, but of course that only covers this summer, and not the rest of my life. I'm writing all that down in longhand first to make sure I'm saying everything that I want to. Then I'll dictate it into a recording machine, so that the typist I choose can take away my tapes and type them up.

Late in the evening Ken comes back, as arranged, to lock the French windows for me. Then he remakes my bed, which Maggie and I can't wait to get into.

Friday, 12 August

I sleep more soundly, probably because I feel safer with the French windows secure. My body doesn't ache so much today.

I've just read in my *Daily Mail* that the Government would like to encourage cancer patients to speak out and dispel the secrecy surrounding the disease. There are so many women like me, and the number will increase as the scheme for efficient screening gets into its stride. Maybe I can be of help to them – I won't mind people knowing what I've been through once I'm strong and back to normal. Over the past decade women have learnt to speak up for themselves. They have developed their talents and shown their strength and determination both mentally and physically. Together we will beat this wretched disease.

Punctually at twelve o'clock, the audio typist I liked the sound of most arrives. She seems a very nice, discreet family woman, and she hasn't recognized me, which is a help. Discretion is as much a priority as typing skill. She will learn a lot about me in the next few months, and I'm determined to keep my secret until I'm ready to tell it.

As time goes on, people are wondering why I'm still not available, and think I'm taking rather too much holiday this summer. Being ill over a holiday period, however, has its advantages, since many companies and employers would quite expect an agent to reply that one was away for at least part of the time.

My bookings are coming through for October, November, December and January, including some of the one hundred charity work-outs for Help the Aged. It's an excellent spur to getting better and regaining, if possible, my original peak of fitness.

Saturday, 13 August

Six weeks to the day, and I feel quite good. Mr Scott said I would make my recovery in six to eight weeks, and it seems he was right. I'm happy, more comfortable and confident this morning, and with Peter here by my side for the weekend I begin to feel more like my old self. We make love this morning, though still with great hesitancy. Peter's so nervous he'll hurt me when we cuddle, and in truth I can't relax completely in case he does. I still have to be careful stretching my arms up or out, but the never-ending presence of my far from sexy corset is a constant reprimand.

I decide I'll face the shopping centre this morning. I've all sorts of bits and pieces to buy. Peter would prefer to go on his own and get everything done at top speed. I sense his irritation, but explain I'm feeling like a caged bird wanting to spread its wings. For my sake, he cools down.

It irritates me that I'm still dependent and haven't quite got up enough courage to drive again. I'm nervous in case I get into traffic difficulties and have to move quickly, which might pull at the wounds. I don't want to jeopardize my recovery, which

I want to be one hundred per cent successful. I feel grateful I've been given this second chance, and I'm going to hang on to it with all the strength, both mental and physical, I can muster. To throw away this second bite at the apple – to disturb the work of skilful surgeons and to disregard the care and understanding of my close friends and relatives – would be absurd.

After a beer and sandwich on the quay I sleep away the afternoon in preparation for my first social event away from my close circle of protective friends. We've been invited to a barbecue at the golf club by neighbours Janet and John Oliver. Although they know I've been ill, they don't know I've had cancer. It's a nice gathering, but I'm thankful to be sitting down for most of the evening. By eleven o'clock I've had enough, and gracefully we make our exit.

Sunday, 14 August

I've always been a bad sleeper, but this is getting ridiculous. I wake at 1.30, the cat joins me, and we spend many sleepless hours talking to each other in the spare room. As the sun comes up I finally fall asleep. Peter decides to leave me in bed dozing, and eventually brings me a very late breakfast in bed.

He wants to get on, so he cycles down to his mother's and visits various other friends, calling in at the local hostelry on his way back. He deserves some time with the boys.

We spend the rest of the day quietly absorbed in the six Sunday papers we regularly read. But I don't feel good and have a headache. Once again, I think I've overdone it. Nature is telling me to cool down.

Monday, 15 August

A slightly better night – I resorted to a painkiller, which made me feel more comfortable and better able to sleep. I wake up determined to have a good day. With Peter back in London I get on with the domestic chores, but with a little less attack than last week.

I'm living in tracksuits most of the time, with a high-necked cotton vest on over my corset to disguise it. Tee-shirts and sweat shirts are OK if the neck is high and round. My shirts, buttoned up high at the neck, are fine so long as they're of thick enough material not to see through. My newly adapted corset is good under a sundress or swimsuit – but not for long, as I know I need the support of the full corset. My breasts are beginning to feel a little more comfortable each day, but one is still very bruised.

From my window I can see my neighbour Douglas sailing with his grandchildren, who have come to stay for a few days. He's not able to get out very often because his wife is an invalid. Like a small boy, he's thrilled to be out in his boat again. I, too, want to sail, windsurf and ride my bike again – and I'm determined I soon will.

Tuesday, 16 August

The weather continues to be wonderful. I get organized this morning to have Peter's daughter, Holly, to stay for the week. He picks her up in Winchester after driving down from London in the early evening. After supper in the garden, we collect Freda, Peter's mother, and drive to the Bournemouth International Centre, where comedian Michael Barrymore is topping the variety show. I recall working with him in 1983 when, to my delight, I had been invited to perform in front of the Queen.

To appear in two Royal Command performances was a tremendous thrill. On the first occasion it was my honour to open the second half of what must be the most tense and exciting variety show on earth. After a great deal of rehearsal in the Elephant Room, under the stage of the Drury Lane Theatre, we finally got it right. With precise timing, I put the British Olympic gymnastic team through a polished, choreographed routine which built up to a riot of movement, music and colour.

For the line-up I decided against my green leotard and tights in which I had appeared during the show. I asked Frank Usher, the fashion house whose evening dresses I love, to make me a special gown – one of that season's designs, but in slinky green satin. It was a one-shouldered affair, simply draped and reminiscent of a Grecian goddess. I felt so proud that evening as I was presented to the Queen, and again next morning when highlights from the show, including my moment, were shown on Breakfast Time.

The second time was at the Victoria Palace Theatre. Two dozen or so glamorous female personalities were to support Howard Keel, Clayton Farlowe of Dallas, *whilst he sang 'Girls, girls, girls'. The timing and pacing were all-important. At rehearsals, dressed in jeans and easy gear, we were relaxed. We each moved to a spot on the stairs – a bit of a squeeze – then elegantly down and on to an individual dance with Howard Keel. Finally we got into our positions for the line-up and chorus. There wasn't a lot of room for mistakes, and we didn't rehearse in costume. Dress for the occasion was left to our individual choice, but was to be strictly black or white.*

I borrowed a slinky silk number from designer Bruce Oldfield, and – not least for practical reasons – most girls chose to look similarly slim and elegant. But to my irritation I found myself between the only two crinolines – a huge black affair worn by actress Susan Hampshire, and a frothy white number on entertainer Bonnie Langford. I had to fight for my space that night, but it made me walk tall.

Wednesday, 17 August

Peter's so happy to have Holly here with him. They go off windsurfing together and I relax in the garden. Roy comes to help me with the weeding and Ken with the housework. In the early evening David calls. Tides, winds and weather in general can cause mooring chains to disappear into the mud, and David's seems to have done a bunk. We all don our wellies and, whilst the tide is out, walk in the harbour to hunt for it. Mission completed, new chain and buoy attached, we tidy up and Rhonda joins us at the Indian restaurant.

Thursday, 18 August

The weather does the dirty on us, so Peter and Holly go off to shop in Bournemouth. Usually, when Holly's with us, I'm happy to join in and have fun. But this time I feel inadequate, and observe rather than participate. I lose Peter to Holly and feel insecure, but Peter, sensing my insecurity, gives me a look that says it all. *Of course* he loves me, but today is Holly's day, and after all he doesn't see her very often. He's quite right. I've had a lot of support from him, but for the next few days I must take a back seat.

Friday, 19 August

I can't sleep, and I'm frightened of getting back into the rat race. I feel frustrated, feeble and sorry for myself. It all seems to have been so cruel and unnecessary. I wish my brother had made contact with me again. I so hoped he would.

Saturday, 20 August

Seven weeks today. Yet another fight with insomnia, but I will not give in to sleeping pills. It's all too easy to become addicted to them.

It's a busy day. Holly has invited a girlfriend from school for the day. And at breakfast-time, Tim telephones to say he has arrived at RAF Brize Norton in Oxfordshire from Canada. He asks if he and his girlfriend Jill can come for the weekend.

So it's a full house. I'm delighted to see Tim again, and I naturally resume my role of mother. I hope he feels I'm back on form. Everyone has fun throughout the day, but as I grow more tired I get miffed I can't keep up. With everyone out of the house I slip back to bed for the afternoon.

Early evening, we set off to La Mama's, our local favourite Italian restaurant. Roy and his wife Deen join us. We have a great time, and Tim recounts his Canadian experiences. Supper over, we walk *en masse* into Christchurch and head for the sailing club, where we watch the annual Christchurch Regatta firework display. It's nice for me to have Tim and Jill around, and Peter is so happy with Holly. I feel life is getting back to normal.

Sunday, 21 August

Another hectic day. In the morning we enjoy a drink or two with family and friends in the bar of the Avonmouth Hotel, which many Mudeford people regard as their local. The weather is nice again and I'm on form, so we invite a few friends back to the garden, where we barbecue for eleven. At 2.30 Judy, my chum from HTV, arrives from Bristol, as invited, but much later than expected. Her car broke down.

After lunch, all the young and able disappear off to the harbour for an afternoon's boating. I feel upset that I have been automatically left out of these plans, but act the happy hostess to the older guests left. When they leave I decide to go to bed, feeling by now over-tired and in a bad mood.

Later, when I do get up, I find the 'youngsters' have returned but most of them are sound asleep in the lounge, exhausted from their afternoon at sea. I tiptoe back to bed but Peter, hearing me, follows me upstairs and tells me it's bad form to do so. His words sound a bit callous, but I know what he means. We don't get to see the family that often, and he knows I'd be devastated if I fell asleep and found them all gone when I awoke. Besides, he's well aware that I cheer up in the company of those I love.

So I force myself to come down again and act bright until I

can reasonably escape back to bed. There's been so much going on today, and I haven't quite had the energy to cope. I stifle my tears with my pillow so the family, having fun downstairs, can't hear me.

Monday, 22 August

I feel miserable. Tim and Jill have gone on their way and Judy has just left to film in the Wylye valley near Salisbury.

Twenty minutes later Judy phones to say she's broken down again. She has called the RAC already and is waiting for them to come. Peter and Holly decide to go to her rescue and find her at the side of the road, in the company of three New Forest Rangers. She's also managed to lock herself out of the car.

A passing motorist stops and offers to help; he gets the slightly opened window down further. Judy reaches in to release the catch, but in doing so she gets her arm stuck. Just in time, the RAC arrive. In convoy, they all drive to a garage in Christchurch but are told the repair can't be done immediately.

To everyone's surprise Judy now decides she'll buy another car, saying she's been meaning to change for a long time. She finds a secondhand one that suits her down to the ground, but discovers she'll have to hire a third car for the day to get to work, since she can't drive the new one until the insurance and tax have been sorted out.

A man from the garage takes her into town to arrange finance through her building society. He drops her in the High Street. Then, to Judy's horror, she discovers she's lost her building society pass book, which she knows she had at the garage. The driver returns to find her standing in a daze.

To Judy's relief they find the pass book in the back of the car and, finance organized, she returns to the garage to complete her purchase. By now it's lunch-time. She returns to Mudeford and rearranges her filming commitments by telephone.

Holly and Peter, in the meantime, have gone windsurfing. Over a quick snack lunch in the garden we all giggle at the events of the morning.

Finally on our own again, Peter, Holly and I decide to drive into Bournemouth to see *Crocodile Dundee Two*, followed by supper in Christchurch.

Tuesday, 23 August

Holly is up early. Giles, her boyfriend, is arriving for the day, and she and Peter meet him at Christchurch Station. The two teenagers take themselves off for a long walk, up to the quay, over the ferry, along the sandbank and up and over Hengistbury Head. On their return, the tide is right for sailing. I'm not up to joining in all the activity but Peter does, although he's loath to admit he's exhausted and finds it difficult to keep up with the pace set by Holly and Giles!

During the afternoon Annie phones to tell me a journalist in Sussex has been enquiring about my health. He's doing a piece on the forthcoming pantomime in Bognor Regis; having discovered I've pulled out, he wants to know why. Annie has been very tactful, telling him, quite honestly, that I have a personal – female – problem. She would prefer he didn't write about it, so as not to embarrass me. I do hope that's the end of it.

Wednesday, 24 August

It's the end of Holly's holiday with us and Peter drives her back to Winchester. Colin from the World of Sport agency, with whom I work occasionally, telephones to ask me if I can do a two-week cruise on the *QE2*, starting this coming weekend. Obviously someone's fallen out, and Colin doesn't know I've been unwell. I'm flattered, but know I can't, because it would entail taking passengers through daily keep-fit sessions. I've done it before on both the *QE2* and the *Canberra*. Both were wonderful experiences, and I'm sorry to have to turn down the job.

On the previous occasion I was invited to join a QE2 cruise, I accepted the offer with pleasure – I had been working on Breakfast Time *for a year without a break. A week before I was due to go, my editor laughingly told me the BBC had ways of ruining my holiday. Breakfast Time had been given permission to go aboard the QE2 with a film crew for a week to make five programme pieces.*

So what should have been a restful time turned out to be extremely arduous. Often we were up hours before the guests, filming in the kitchens or from the bridge. Another time we filmed throughout the night, reporting as the ship's daily newspaper was written and printed. And on yet another occasion we were down in the bowels of the ship, in the laundry. During the day, with the doctor and the entertainment staff, we made reports on life aboard. One morning I started the programme standing on the bow of the great ship, a lonely figure swinging exercise clubs in the early morning mist.

It was a memorable trip, but the day the BBC crew left I took to my bed with a sore throat. I relaxed, recharged my batteries, and after a day was up and about enjoying my second week without them.

Gary, my contact for the Ford house magazine, *Front Desk*, phones regarding the first of the articles I'm writing for them. He needs copy and pictures by September. We fix a date for the photographic session and I decide to start doing some general exercises in earnest. I feel flabby with so much inactivity, and my body is out of tune. I resolve to start dieting. I've been eating well, perhaps a little too well, with all the fresh food and garden produce. I've even given way to the occasional chocolate and cream. But I've felt my body needed all the good food it could get, and I didn't want to waste essential energy on too much exercise until now. I've been doing plenty of neck, shoulder, arm and back exercises in an attempt to regain my mobility and posture. But now it's time to take my whole body in hand.

After a short trip to the shops in Highcliffe, Peter encourages me to take the wheel of his car to drive home. Even though it's an automatic, with power-assisted steering, I'm apprehensive to begin with – it's the first time I've driven since I went into hospital. However, it feels good to be back behind the wheel again, and I happily drive the few miles to Mudeford.

Thursday, 25 August

Peter's up and off to London by 5.30, and I relax back into domesticity with a sigh of relief. With all the visitors gone, I can now take it more quietly and concentrate my energies on my complete recovery.

I begin exercising, starting, as I always do, with a complete body stretch. I gradually work down from head to toe, concentrating on various muscle groups. Then I pop out to the shops and stock the fridge with low-fat milk, masses of fruit and vegetables, yogurt, fresh fish, nuts and pulses.

Excitedly I keep answering the phone to Annie, who calls regarding work. It would appear it's all coming back.

Any spare time I have, I concentrate on writing the linking passages for my book. I'm glad now that I took Peter's advice to make a detailed diary entry each day. By publishing my diary as part of the book, and telling the truth about my past few months, I realize I run the risk of turning away potential clients. They may regard me as not having a healthy image any more. It's ironic, because in fact I'm very well. It's being so fit and strong that has enabled me to recuperate so quickly.

Friday, 26 August

Work continues to pour in as I get ready for a weekend away in Warwickshire. But the doorbell stops me, and I find Marion and Pete have returned from their two months away in Spain. They look tanned and well, but I learn Pete has been out of sorts. However, a Spanish specialist seems to have temporarily sorted him out. Batchy, our fisherman friend and coxswain of the Mudeford lifeboat, sees us in the window as he drives past, so he pops in. We chatter away exchanging news, which includes talk of two local women who have been found to have breast cancer. I stay very quiet.

Saturday, 27 August

Eight weeks ago today since the operation, and who would have believed I would feel so well? We make an early start and, though it's bank holiday weekend, find the journey not too bad. We book into our hotel and go off to visit the Town and Country Festival at Stoneleigh. Richard, my producer from Central TV, has told me that advance copies of *Look Good, Feel Great* are out and will be on sale in the Healthy Living exhibition at the Festival. He's involved in the administration, and has asked me to call in to see him if I feel fit enough.

The vast showground, home of the Royal Show, is a hive of activity with people from Birmingham, Coventry and surrounding areas packing in on this sunny weekend. We soon find the Healthy Living exhibition, where I'm delighted to see members of the Keep Fit Association with their teacher, Joan, who will be doing demonstrations throughout the day.

An attractive woman in her thirties comes up and asks if I remember her. Looking closely, I recall that she and I had worked together with Christopher as models at some of the large fashion presentations, including the Leather Fair, held at the National Exhibition Centre in Birmingham many years ago. Sue now runs the local model agency, and today puts on a spectacular fashion show. Her models are beautiful and well groomed, and she must be very proud of them. Another face seems familiar and I realize one of her girls was the teenage model who had been part of my team all those years ago. As I watch the girls going through their paces, I suddenly feel older.

Sunday, 28 August

Time for a little more sightseeing today, including a visit to Coventry and the cathedral, with its dramatic, multi-coloured stained glass windows and high vaulted roof supported by fine columns. The organ pipes are so impressive and I'm sorry not to be able to hear their sound – unfortunately we're between services. I adore organ music, and mentally earmark the cathedral for another visit – perhaps for an organ recital.

Monday, 29 August

We check out of the hotel and decide to go back to Stoneleigh, which is on our way home. At the Healthy Living exhibition crowds are gathering in anticipation of the keep-fit demonstration. I'm delighted to see Brian 'Killer' Kilcline in the crowd, which isn't difficult. The captain of Coventry City's FA Cup-winning team stands six foot two, and with his reputation on the field it's easy to see how he came by his nickname.

In the last series he was my unwilling guinea pig, but a tremendous sport. I well remember the press call we did at the Coventry City ground. After staging the usual promotional shots, I suggested we stood back to back and linked arms. I encouraged Brian to bend forward, lifting me on to his back, as I kicked my legs high into the air. It made sensational pictures. But there was a better one to come as Brian lost his balance and I, in self-defence, hurled him to the ground. It was hilarious, but he hasn't forgiven me. My other guinea pig was actor Tony Adams from *Crossroads*, who, having trained in ballet, was an excellent pupil.

The music for the demonstration begins and is infectious. Soon I feel myself moving and swaying in time to it. Before we know it, both Brian and I are participating. I can see Peter looking at me apprehensively, but I know my body well enough and feel everything is under control. As the tempo ups it's time for me to stop, but I'm exhilarated and realize I will soon be able to enjoy an exercise session again. But I'm nervous in case 'Killer' decides to take his revenge on me, and move away quickly. The crowds queue for autographs and I feel back on top of the world.

On the way home I'm a bit tired but pleased with myself, and Peter's pleased for me too. I feel a page has been turned.

Tuesday, 30 August

Each day now I feel that little bit stronger, and I'm able to tackle more of the domestic chores. Up and down the three flights of stairs in this little house, although tiring, is helping to build up my stamina. My problem has been finding the right balance between activity and adequate rest. I should do as I teach – listen to my body, and when it complains, stop.

I'd like to be driving more but find my own car, a Mazda RX7, too heavy for me. I decide to leave driving it for a few more weeks, but it does make me walk more, which must be doing me good. That car has been my pride and joy since I began on *Breakfast Time*. I had seen the model some years previously in America, where it was very popular. So with a little extra money in my pocket I had spoilt myself and bought one.

Later the same year I was asked to work at the Motor Show in Birmingham – not with small cars, but with huge trucks. On the Renault stand I invited truckers and visitors to join me and do themselves a service by switching on their own engines and looking after their bodywork. Our keep-fit sessions caught the attention of the public, press and television, and Renault did marvellous business.

Wednesday, 31 August

Clare, my childhood friend whom I last saw at Henley Regatta, drives down from Weybridge in Surrey to see me. The weather is fine, so we decide to walk to the quay and catch the ferry to the sandbank. We stroll in the sun and have a simple lunch in the café overlooking the harbour. Fortified, we walk on up the rough-hewn steps at the end of Hengistbury Head and climb to the top, where we sit amongst the heather and enjoy the magnificent view. To our left we can see as far as the Needles off the Isle of Wight, and to our right past Bournemouth Bay and on to Lulworth Cove. I feel puffed after all those steps, and realize I'm still out of condition.

Having caught my breath, we descend the steps and walk around the Head and on to an area of beach which summer visitors don't often find. A lot of work has been done constructing new groynes during the winter, and lovely little beaches of fine sand have since formed.

Clare declares her hand. It appears I've walked her off her feet and she's got blisters on her heels. We sit down and, since she's not wearing socks, I give her mine. A little more comfortably we walk back and catch the ferry home.

But I've got the bit between my teeth now and, determined to show Clare the area, take her into Christchurch. We walk around the gardens and grounds of the medieval Christchurch Priory, over the little bridge by the water mill and on to the sailing club, where we sit and take in the view. Back home she collapses in exhaustion and we laugh over a cup of tea. But at least one of us feels fit and fine.

SEPTEMBER

Thursday, 1 September

Seems like summer's disappeared. Gale-force winds in the night have blown open the garden shed, which looks in danger of falling apart. Still in my dressing-gown, and with difficulty, I tie it together. When Ken, my Man Thursday, arrives his first job will be to make it secure.

My breasts are hurting me a lot today, which worries me. But as I dress after my morning bath I realize the elastic in my corset has become weak through constant washing and the effects of the calendula ointment. I'm scared that the lack of support will set me back. I can't afford to take any chances, so I lie back on the sofa and read for the day, which makes me more comfortable and relieves the strain. Perhaps yesterday's exercising was too much for me and I'm in need of stronger elastic. I must call Mr Crosswell and get Peter to bring me down a new corset tomorrow.

The papers are full of radio broadcaster Ray Moore's brave fight against cancer. I cast my mind back to the Royal Tournament of last year, and the press luncheon in particular. With Ray and his wife we shared a glass or two of champagne, seemingly without a care in the world. Who could have guessed that within the year we would both be facing the challenge of cancer? My thoughts this morning are with Ray and his devoted wife Alma.

Friday, 2 September

I'm still anxious about this recurrence of pain. Did I walk too much with Clare on Wednesday? But I'd felt so well and enjoyed myself, thinking I was back on form. I do hope it's just the elastic. The front of my corset is now very saggy and limp so I put it on back to front, which is difficult because it means the zip is now at the back. I decide that the spare one, worn on top the right way round, may help support me even more. What a comical sight I look!

Without further ado I telephone Mr Crosswell's assistant and ask her to look out another corset for me and to send it round to Peter's office on a bike, so he can bring it down when he returns to Dorset tonight. I ask the girl to put it in a parcel addressed to him and marked 'Personal'. I giggle at the thought of his staff opening the packet, seeing the corset and suspecting Peter of a secret they shouldn't know about!

When he arrives at seven o'clock I put the new corset on with some relief. Immediately I'm more comfortable and feel less pain. Under control again, we set off to have supper out in Paw-Paw's restaurant in Highcliffe with our neighbours Janet and John. I find it easy to ignore the past two months and get on with the present when I'm with people who don't know the truth.

Saturday, 3 September

The pain is still niggling away and I cancel plans to go out again tonight. Should I be resting more, or do I need more exercise? I sit writing my book quietly, but find I'm stiffening up and the wounds are pulling. As rest isn't working I decide to go for a walk.

Peter and I catch the bus to Highcliffe, where we step out smartly through the village and on down to the cliff edge. A steep descent takes us to the long, pebbly beach. The fresh sea breeze streams through our hair and makes us catch our breath.

Halfway along the beach I need a rest and sit on a ledge of pebbles in the warm autumn sunshine, staring out to sea. We watch the waves crash and ripple up the beach, which is quiet and deserted. Most of the holidaymakers have gone home, and we've got it to ourselves again. We throw pebbles into the sea, making them skim and dance across the water.

With a fresh burst of energy we walk on to Avon Beach where we stop and buy ice-creams. Licking the cones like two small children we wander on to Mudeford quay and watch other, smaller, children crouching down eagerly with their crab lines and buckets. We inspect their day's catch of tiny crabs.

Sunday, 4 September

I feel really good this morning – better for the exercise, a good night's sleep and the added support of my new corset. It's a nice lazy day, but as the afternoon draws on we sadly pack up our belongings, pop Maggie into her box and return to the flat.

Monday, 5 September

Back in London a cold nip in the air signals the return of autumn. I reorganize my wardrobe, bringing forward my thicker woollen clothes and tucking my thin, cool cottons away. Dressed smartly, I get ready to see Mr Scott and Mr Crosswell at the Royal Marsden.

The taxi driver asks my destination and enquires what I will be doing there. I reply I'm visiting people. Sadly, he tells how he has recently lost his wife, after thirty-one years of happy marriage, as a result of breast cancer. He tells me she had left it too late. She had felt lumps each month in her breast, but thought it was just a symptom of her periods. When eventually she asked him to feel the lumps one of them was very large indeed. Within days of seeing her doctor she had a mastectomy, but it was too late and the cancer had already spread throughout her body.

I sense that talking like this is helping him. He goes on to tell me that breast cancer and the subsequent mastectomy is the worst thing, to his mind, that can happen to a woman. Women say they don't mind, he says, but they do really. He is clearly very distressed at the memory of his wife's suffering. I listen to him quietly, knowing only too well how right he is.

At the hospital they're happy with my progress, and although one breast isn't in quite such good shape as the other, they hope in time it will right itself. I tell them I'm working and exercising again – my only problem is I have to be photographed at the end of the month in my green leotard and tights, and I don't have two nipples. Amused, they ask me if I frequent sex shops. 'Certainly not!' I reply. They ask me if Peter does, and I tell them I don't think so. It's a pity, because apparently false nipples are sold in these places! However, they promise to put me in touch with a nurse who will supply me with a stick-on model as a temporary measure.

I ask when I will be able to have the operation to reconstruct my nipple. After a close inspection they say it is far too early. I had hoped to have it done by Christmas, but they tell me it would be better to leave it till later, when everything will have settled down. Jokingly, both surgeons conclude I shan't have a new nipple for Christmas but I can have it for Easter instead.

Mr Crosswell comments that I will be able to share a nipple. I look confused. He tells me he will be able to take half of my existing right nipple to make a nipple for my left breast. To reconstruct an areola, he will take skin from my groin. This shouldn't prove painful, and may be performed under a local anaesthetic. The mind boggles.

Tuesday, 6 September

Ian performs his monthly magic and gets my hair back in order so that I can pick up where I left off months ago. I travel into the West End to see Annie and talk about work. I feel in good form. A client is to meet me at the office to discuss some future business, but as she's been delayed Annie suggests I pop out for an hour or so.

I walk down to Oxford Street, but the weather is hot and the crowds unbearable, and soon I begin to feel uncomfortable. I'm not ready to charge around with my usual energy and, somewhat deflated, I return to Annie's office and sip tea. The client wants me to write a small book on a specific feminine problem which will need a lot of research. I agree, although I know it will be hard work completing it in the required time. What a lot of writing I will have done this year.

I'm weary when I meet Peter for a lift home, and I'm not amused by talk of his high-flying acquaintances, their expensive cars and fancy lifestyles. Acidly I remark, 'Who cares about their new-found material wealth? It's of no importance – it's just a load of bullshit.' How cancer makes one's priorities crystal-clear and cuts through the nonsense surrounding poseurs! I'm in a bad temper, but know I'm just over-tired. London is exhausting and I've overdone it, but fortunately Peter realizes this and takes it all quite philosophically.

Wednesday, 7 September

I feel better for a good night's sleep, and start putting stuff together for Mudeford tomorrow.

I travel into Peter's office, where I'm to meet an acquaintance to discuss the possibility of yet more work in the literary field – this time a book for children. As I walk into the office for the first time in months I'm embarrassed to meet his staff. Knowing my secret, they must be looking me up and down, and I feel ridiculously self-conscious. However the book idea, generated quite unintentionally some months ago over the dinner table, gets taken a stage further.

Then I walk down to the Meridien Hotel in Piccadilly, which houses Champneys luxurious health club in its basement. I'm going to meet my fairy godmother, Elizabeth. It's good to see her again under normal circumstances, looking radiant as ever. Like two excited schoolgirls we sit down and chatter for hours. I owe her so much.

Pleased with my progress and her approval, I take myself off for an appointment with Liz Calder. We firm up details for my book, and I enjoy the feeling of being back in the swing of things.

Thursday, 8 September

A call on my answerphone has given me details of a casting being held this morning at a dance studio in Putney. The weather's turned very hot again and I don't really have the time to attend, as I've planned to pick up Dorothy in Bristol at lunch-time to take her to Mudeford for a few days. But nothing ventured, nothing gained.

I set off early, looking bright and breezy in my Florida tracksuit, but when I get there I see I'm in the wrong clothes. The large, mirrored studio is full of exquisitely dressed models. My model agent has failed to tell me to be dressed this smartly, and I feel at a disadvantage as I'm put through my paces. They're looking for a team of good movers, attractive men and women who will appear in a video and photographs for Saab cars. Loud music blares as groups of us are instructed to step forward, to the side, back, turn, hold it for a count of four and so on. Wearing my Reeboks, I feel as if I've got two left feet. I'm confused, out of step and out of time. I've lost my confidence and, not surprisingly, the job.

Hurriedly I leave the studio, but turn as somebody calls my name. It's actress Rula Lenska, a friend who looks blooming, which makes me feel worse. She tells me she's rehearsing Noël Coward's *Blithe Spirit*, which is to open soon in Bromley and then go on tour. I tell her I've just fluffed a casting. She understands, knowing that in our business we win some and lose some.

I step out briskly to walk the fair distance back home to Battersea to rid myself of the frustration. I've a long way to go to reach the peak of that particular profession, if ever again.

I pack the car and apprehensively drive the hundred or so miles to Bristol. It's my first long drive since the operation, and by the time I reach Dorothy I'm thankful to stop. I feel a bit uncomfortable across my chest, but after a short rest the two of us drive on to Frome in Somerset. It's a little off our route, but it enables me to visit my cousin Mary.

She comes to the door with her three lovely little girls, aged four, three and eighteen months. It's lovely to see them all – they seem such a contented family and the girls are so charming and well behaved.

Tea refreshes us, but I'm relieved when Dorothy and I eventually arrive in Mudeford.

Friday, 9 September

In the garden, Dorothy and I relax and reminisce. After lunch we drive to the local garden centre and buy a few plants, which I put in on our return. Over a well-deserved cup of tea, I sit back and admire the results.

Batchy calls with a fishy present. He follows me into the kitchen where, much to Dorothy's amusement, he asks for a large, sharp knife and demonstrates how to prepare a lobster *properly*. He obviously doesn't think I do it right! Peter is welcomed home by the smell of fresh fish which very soon disappears, leaving us all, including Maggie, licking our lips and well satisfied.

Saturday, 10 September

I land another fish this morning. Roy has had another successful week salmon fishing and knows we're very appreciative fish-lovers. The weather's good, so Peter wants to go sailing. Dorothy and I, on the other hand, decide to take the day nice and easy – we've been invited to tea by Lala, who is staying with her new baby in Sopley in the New Forest, just a few miles away.

Returning home at the appointed hour, I'm surprised to find Peter absent. After two hours I start to worry. But, windswept and laughing, he returns and regales us with boating tales, having spent a hilarious afternoon with David. Running out of petrol off the Isle of Wight, they had to act quickly to get fuel to enable them to return at all tonight. He changes his clothes, and we meet up with David and his wife Rhonda for an evening at the Indian restaurant.

Sunday, 11 September

I cook the salmon in foil with grapes and fresh parsley for lunch. It tastes delicious.

With Dorothy resting in the garden, Peter and I get fuelled with determination and dig out two small fir trees, casualties of last October's hurricane. But halfway through the tough operation I decide to take it easy, knowing I'm not as strong as I'd thought. It's odd, at this stage, what I can and can't do. One of the hardest jobs is plugging the flex into the back of the electric kettle. It seems a simple task, and yet it uses muscles that still aren't up to such demands.

Peter has arranged for Dorothy to have a lift back to Bristol to spare me the drive, and she leaves us after tea. It's been a good weekend. I've enjoyed having her to stay and the change of scenery has been good for her.

Suddenly there's a resounding bang as the maroons go off, calling the lifeboatmen and helpers in the village to their action stations. A yachtsman or windsurfer is probably in trouble at sea. Peter and I run quickly down to the end of the quay to the lifeboat station. The launchers speedily handle the Atlantic 21 lifeboat into the water as the crew clamber into their gear and adjust their equipment. The twenty-two-foot rigid inflatable boat and the three crewmen are ready in minutes, and are soon off at high speed.

Monday, 12 September

After a good night's sleep, I feel really well this morning. I drive forty miles to Chris Dunning's Hampshire home for a lunch-time meeting of a fund-raising committee. We're raising money for Salisbury Cathedral's SOS (Save Our Spire) appeal, and because of my showbusiness and fashion background Chris has asked me to co-operate on a fund-raising Evening of Fashion to be held next month in Salisbury's City Hall. The ancient cathedral with its magnificent spire is in need of repair because the stone has weathered and eroded over the centuries. Over £6.5 million is urgently required for the necessary work, to be completed over the next ten years. The appeal is headed by Prince Charles, who is taking a personal interest.

As I drive home, stimulated by the meeting and with my head full of ideas, I know I'm getting back to normal.

Tuesday, 13 September

Derek and Audrey drive the difficult cross-country route from Stoke St Gregory in Somerset to visit me for the day. I'm so pleased to see them, and give them a conducted tour of the village. At lunch-time we land up in the Avonmouth Hotel where I introduce them to the locals. We linger over the excellent traditional English meal, admiring the harbour view and watching the wildlife.

Back in the house and on my own again, I come across my exercise clubs and take them into the garden where there's room for me to swing them. I find the movement good for loosening the tension that has built up in my neck and shoulders and across my back. The exercise improves my posture and works on the muscles across my chest and under my arms. I breathe deeply and swing rhythmically, and it feels good.

Wednesday, 14 September

It's four months since my cancer was diagnosed. It's a sad truth that, once other people know of your problem, you discover many friends and acquaintances have also experienced cancer. I've just learnt of the recent death from brain cancer of the husband of a fellow-model and great friend of mine, Pam Gingell, after thirty-eight years of marriage. And in Mudeford Marion and Pete have heard the devastating news that their middle daughter, Julie, aged twenty-one, has leukaemia.

I make a date to go and see the doctor at the Amarant Centre again. I owe him so much for that early diagnosis, and must thank him personally.

Thursday, 15 September

I find writing is therapeutic, and in any case I have to do it now whilst my mind is sharp and uncluttered with everyday trivia. In a few months' time I will probably be too busy. As I write I sort out the muddle I call my life and put it into perspective. My hopes and fears, my priorities and ambitions all begin to fit into place.

Friday, 16 September

A letter from my producer at Central TV, Richard Patching, tells me there is an added uncertainty regarding the transmission dates and time slots for the new series of Look Good, Feel Great. I'm fed up with the number of changes which have been made over the past few months, and wonder whether the programme will be shown at all.

Peter is coming down from London today but will go straight to the Boat Show in Southampton, where he'll meet up with friends to look around. The weather's so good it inspires me to take myself off to the garden centre again to buy masses of colourful winter pansies. I then spend a lovely day weeding, digging, pulling out and planting in. It's my most energetic day yet. I sweep the paths and water in the new plants, tidy up the garden and prepare for the autumn.

I'm pleased with the work I've been able to accomplish and sit down tired but satisfied. On Peter's return, I greedily go along with his suggestion of fish and chips for supper.

Saturday, 17 September

Not surprisingly, the whole of my body aches this morning as a result of yesterday's strenuous activity. But I know it's normal, and decide on more exercise to rid myself of the stiffness. We walk to Southbourne, to look at the work being done to the cliff edge and beach. A large vessel full of pipes and platforms is at anchor off the beach. It's the 1500 ton dredger *James Ensor*, and one of its pipes is attached to a huge floating pipeline in the sea. The pipeline leads to a T-junction of more enormous pipes which lie along the beach. The vessel has previously sucked up shingle from the continental shelf, which now comes gushing out with tremendous force to refurbish and build up the shoreline.

Along with others out for an afternoon stroll, we stand high up on the windy cliff edge watching this fascinating procedure. I ask one of the workmen how long it will all take. Apparently it's a month's work to replenish the eroded beach, and the pipeline will be gradually extended along the shoreline as required. We observers are most impressed and look forward to enjoying the beautiful beaches next year.

Richard and Sue from America are down in the area visiting relations. Sue is now four and a half months pregnant and looks very well. The four of us have a lot to chatter about over supper tonight.

Sunday, 18 September

Sue calls round in the morning for coffee while the men take themselves off to discuss business. She's surprised to find me so fit. I assure her I feel very well, and even find it difficult myself to believe that so much has happened since my Florida trip.

Later Peter and I take ourselves over on the ferry to the sandbank to join David and Rhonda's lunch-time gathering. We're late-comers to what has probably been the last of the season's barbecues. Several other people from the village have the same idea, and as the sun sets it finds a dozen of us in deckchairs on the beach, relaxing in its long shadows.

The last ferry has gone and David offers us a lift back to Christchurch in his boat. It will be my first boat trip this year. Along with Pete and Marion, Peter and I scramble aboard. The boat takes us along the edge of the sandbank where many huts are now shuttered up for winter, their owners having learnt a hard lesson during last October's hurricane.

After the boat has been made secure we drive to Pete's house, where Marion and I prepare lobsters. We're joined for supper by two of their daughters. Julie, the third, sadly can't be there – she's in hospital in Boscombe, where they are doing what they can to treat her leukaemia.

Tired but happy, we finally collapse into bed. It's been a nice weekend.

Monday, 19 September

Refreshed, Peter returns to London for the week and leaves me confidently to fend for myself. My post brings good news. My claim for the hospital and operation fees has been met by my private health scheme. But, as I anticipated, not in full.

An invitation from the Christchurch and Mudeford Venture Scouts asks me to be their guest in a few weeks' time to taste their camp cooking for part of an award scheme. I remember my days as a Brownie and Girl Guide and smile at the thought of our camp suppers. It's lucky I like burnt sausages.

The Regent Community Centre in Christchurch want me to judge their annual Snow Queen competition. The Queen, whom I will crown, will be a young girl of eleven to fifteen, and her two princesses between seven and ten. They will take pride of place on the Chamber of Trade's float in the annual Christmas procession at the beginning of December in aid of local charities.

I enjoy taking part in these events and am pleased to think I can be of help. I reply yes to both invitations.

Tuesday, 20 September

I enjoy the day writing up my diary, together with recollections of my earlier life, for the book. Theresa, my typist, was a good choice, though partly for reasons that sadden me and remind me again what a small world it is. As she brings me the neatly typed copy, she tells me she will be unavailable for a day or so. She hadn't intended to tell me until the book was finished, but this enforced absence has obliged her to let me in on *her* secret. She's going to see a specialist in London, and I'm sorry to learn she too has been battling with cancer for eleven years, since she was just twenty-six. She, herself, helps counsel other cancer sufferers.

Wednesday, 21 September

I got carried away with writing last night and stayed up till 1.30 this morning. I've a sore throat and feel a bit off. I think I've overdone it again and had better take things easy today.

Thursday, 22 September

I'm up early to pack Maggie and myself into the car and drive back to London. Richard and Sue are coming to stay in the flat tonight. The four of us are going to a special performance of John Chapman's farce, *Dry Rot*, at the Lyric Theatre. It's a charity event in aid of the Stars' Organization for Spastics. The actor Brian Rix returns to the West End stage tonight after some years away.

We meet Jan Leeming and her husband Eric in the bar and find we are all sitting together. Jan is pleased to see me back on form. It's a good evening and I'm delighted to see actor Derek Griffiths, my old chum Ebenazar from *Aladdin*, playing the part of Flash Harry so amusingly.

Both Peter and I seem to have developed a heavy cold, but nevertheless enjoy ourselves and go out on the town afterwards with our guests.

Friday, 23 September

I've got a headache and a sore throat and I've lost my voice. At a meeting of the Stars' Organization for Spastics Committee this morning everyone agrees that last night was good, but the response and therefore the profit was not as it should have been due to the postal strike. It appears many charity events have been affected by it. It's such a shame after all the effort and preparation people have put in. I've taken with me some signed copies of my book and record *Get Fit with the Green Goddess*, which I hope the charity can use at other fund-raising events.

I visit Liz Calder during the afternoon to deliver some copy and return home with Peter. We hurriedly change our clothes and drive down to lovely Goodwood House in West Sussex, where we've been invited for a business reception.

Saturday, 24 September

It's twelve weeks today since the operation to rid me of breast cancer. It's been a more difficult exercise, but I've regained my mobility and my energy is returning daily. I've picked up the threads of my life and work is coming in, although I'm restricted in what I can do and fear I may never return to my former level of physical activity. But I feel good in myself and about myself, and I'm optimistic for the future.

I'm still wearing my corset, which keeps me feeling comfortable and secure, but occasionally I leave it off for a few hours when I dress up to go out. I'm doing a quarter of an hour's work-out each day and my body is regaining its tone and strength, but I've yet to build up my stamina.

Peter and I feel very close, and the bond between myself and my boys has been strengthened. But I'm sorry still not to have heard from my brother since his phone calls in June – though I'm too proud to go seeking sympathy from him.

Back in London, I take the opportunity of a lift into the West End and whilst Peter pops into his office I've time to browse. The big stores and shops are full of smart autumn clothes, but I'm not tempted today. The thought of undressing in the communal changing rooms causes me embarrassment. My winter wardrobe will have to wait.

Sunday, 25 September

It's a lovely autumn day and Peter accompanies me to Ham Polo Club at Richmond, where I've been asked as a guest to a charity event in aid of the Royal Marsden Hospital. The match stars National Hunt jockey Bob Champion, who so successfully fought and won his personal battle against cancer some years ago. He looks very well and I congratulate him on the imminent birth of his baby, due in two weeks.

We join a table of personalities for lunch. Actress Lisa Goddard is playing in the match. Actor David Healy is umpiring it. Comedy actor Trevor Bannister provides us with non-stop humour, and TV presenter Angela Rippon, with her great interest in horses, keeps us well informed. Anton Rogers acts as auctioneer. It's a good day, with all the proceeds from the event going towards the hospital's cancer research. Nobody suspects my intense personal interest, but I know that, when the truth is out, I will be able to help much more.

It will soon be time to close my diary. Life's becoming too busy for me to keep it up. Anyway, the purpose for which it was originally begun has been achieved. I'm through all that now, and must look to the future.

The last three months have forced me to stand still. The experience has taught me to be aware and to communicate. Aware of my blessings and priorities, aware of the importance of good health, aware of my own vulnerability and more aware of trivia and insincerity. I've discovered my inner strength and the need to build on it. I've felt the happiness of friendship given and received and the essential inter-dependence of human beings. We all need to communicate, to share our feelings of love, happiness, sadness and compassion, and to spend time listening to others.

From my brush with cancer, I've learnt to think positively. I've gained confidence, self-respect and an inner peace. I feel more strongly than ever before the need to live life for the day, with just a cautious eye to the future. But most of all, I've learnt not to take my blessings for granted, and to thank God I'm alive.

October

Epilogue

Last week, looking for a special occasion dress, I visited Cibi, a small, high-class fashion shop in Beauchamp Place in Knightsbridge. I had left off my corset and, watched by Gina, the owner, who knew nothing of my traumatic summer, I clambered self-consciously in and out of beautiful creations which she had selected for my approval. Zipping me up, she commented now comfortable my new sports bra looked, and I assured her it was. She told me I was a joy to fit and wished all her customers were so easy, adding, 'But then you're so lucky to have such a beautiful figure.'

She didn't realize the truth of her remark or the profound effect her simple compliment had on me. As I stood looking at my reflection I finally appreciated just how lucky I had been I could have hugged her.

A NOTE ON THE AUTHOR

Born in the West Country, Diana Moran now lives in London. Apart from working in television – most recently hosting ITV's *Look Good, Feel Great* – she writes for numerous magazines and newspapers, has made records and cassettes and conducts exercise sessions all over the country. She is the mother of two grown-up sons.